Roz Denny is a London-ba[...] and author of over twe[...] cuisines, including vegeta[...] ...healthy eating. She feels a particular affinity with the subject of weight control for vegetarians, having undergone a dramatic weight loss herself (which she has kept off) and brought up two vegetarian daughters!

THE GREEN DIET

ROZ DENNY

ORION

An Orion Paperback
First published in Great Britain in 2002 by
Orion Books Ltd,
Orion House, 5 Upper St Martin's Lane,
London WC2H 9EA

A CIP catalogue record for this book is available
from the British Library.

ISBN: 0 75281 747 7

Printed and bound in Great Britain by
The Guernsey Press Co. Ltd, Guernsey, C.I.

To Felicity

CONTENTS

INTRODUCTION

There is a myth that vegetarians don't have to worry about their weight. That because they have given up eating meat they are permanently slim. In fact, weight gain has nothing to do with whether one eats meat or not. Omnivores and vegetarians alike can put on too much weight for the same reason: because they eat too much and don't exercise enough. Basically, if we consume more calories than we need, from whatever food source – we will gain weight.

The process of dieting in order to lose weight seems to be very much a phenomenon of the last fifty years. It's ironic that at a time when most of us have access to bountiful supplies of food, we look for ways of cutting back on what we eat. We are also becoming very aware of what we eat. Medical research indicates that many diseases afflicting mankind are diet-related; in other words, we seem to bring them upon ourselves. So it makes sense that if you want to be in control of your food intake, you need to take a little time to become familiar with the ingredients.

The last twenty years or so have seen a number of theme diets come and go. Some of them reassure us that if you follow them for a couple of weeks, then hey presto, like magic a new slim you will emerge. For most of us who have to watch our weight, we clutch at these magic-wand diets with their promises and formulas. Increasingly, waif-like celebrities are used as endorsements with the implication that if you can stick to one or other formula diet, you will somehow acquire a similar glam image.

> *Basically, if we consume more calories than we need, from whatever food source – we will gain weight.*

> *The current eating pattern is increasingly one of solitary grazing, of eating to ward off hunger pangs, eating 'on the run' and snatching snacks.*

We follow charts, plans and theories such as not eating certain foods in combination because they fight in our stomachs, or we fill up with big bowls of low-carb/high-protein soup.

In their way, these diets play their part. Some of us do indeed lose a few kilos (or pounds) but this is more because we are controlling our food intake overall. Then gradually, we slip back into old familiar ways and within a year or so, we are back to breathing in when we zip up our skirts and talking to friends about yet another miracle cure diet.

What is missing from many of these diets is a sense of the real world and why we gain weight in the first place. Before we start trying to slim, we should find out more about our own daily diets. What do we eat that causes us to put on weight? What sort of lifestyles do we follow that dictate our feeding habits? Mealtimes have become of secondary importance to most of us. The current eating pattern is increasingly one of solitary grazing, of eating to ward off hunger pangs, eating 'on the run' and snatching snacks. When we do actually sit down to eat calmly, it is often in a social environment where the general spirit of well-being causes us to shed inhibitions and overindulge. We eat over-rich food, or higher-fat convenience foods, washed down with alcohol or sugary drinks. We gulp and gobble with little thought for the consequences.

All food *per se* does you no harm, unless of course it is obviously poisonous or you are specifically allergic to certain foodstuffs. There is no such thing as a bad food or a bad diet. What determines whether or not we have a weight 'problem' is the amount of certain foods eaten, and whether we use them up in energy immediately or store them as body fat. There are many non-meat foods that can lead to weight storage problems if eaten to excess. Once we have stopped growing upwards, if we consistently eat more calories than we use in energy, we will start to grow outwards.

So – this book is offered on the same principle of teaching a starving man to fish or farm. You aim to feed him for life, not for a week or two. Take a little time to read the information on the nutritional background of your daily food so that you don't repeat the same mistakes of weight gain. Instead of trying to memorize some complicated diet combination, learn about what you eat.

If you know the calorie and fat values of foods and adjust your diet accordingly, once you get back in control and lose your excess weight, you can keep it off. It is simply a question of changing your eating habits and retraining your palate. Even with the occasional blip you can get back on course. Your best equipment is your eyes, your fingers, a full-length mirror and a pair of bathroom scales. I also keep a pair of benchmark jeans. When I have to breathe in to do them up, then it's time to watch it.

There are many non-meat foods that can lead to weight storage problems if eaten to excess.

The aim of this book is to arm you with the facts about foods and to introduce you to ingredients that taste great without piling on the calories. Then no one can ever say good, tasty food is boring. You can be your own master and need never diet as such again.

CHAPTER ONE

So How Overweight Are You?

It is estimated that around a third of us weigh more than is good for us. It is also believed that about half of us are on some diet or other, or are at least 'watching' our weight. Sadly few of us are born with ideally proportioned bodies, or rather what our Western culture perceives as attractive physiques. One only has to look at pictures of 1950s movie stars to see that they would be considered quite well-rounded now compared to the current ultra-thin catwalk 'supermodels' or movie stars, who run the risk of losing new film roles if they look halfway normal. It is surely no coincidence that the advent of the bikini coincided with the appearance of slimming diets in our magazines and beauty pages.

To measure just how overweight you may or may not be, scientists have devised a measure of obesity called the **Body Mass Index** or **BMI**.

HOW TO MEASURE YOUR BMI

Divide your weight in kilos by your height in metres, squared. A healthy BMI figure is between 20 and 25. A BMI of 30 or more is likely to lead to health problems.

For example, I am 57 kilos in weight, and my height is 1.60m, which squared is 2.56. So my BMI is 57 divided by 2.56, which comes to 22.26. This is well within the range for a healthy weight– phew! But I could still consider myself to be a little overweight and feel the need to cut down as long as I didn't diet too seriously and dip below a BMI of 20.

Alternatively you can **'pinch an inch' to check.** Pinch your flesh around your waist or your relaxed biceps or under your armpit. If there is more than 1 inch (2.5cm) of soft fat, then it's time to take control.

YOUR DAILY CALORIE INTAKE

We all use energy simply by being alive – breathing, blinking, even just sitting reading a newspaper. This is known as our **basal metabolic rate**. Then we need additional energy for simple daily chores – housework, shopping, sitting at a desk and thinking. The actual amount will depend on how active we are.

Men generally use 1600 calories a day and women around 1300. But if you want a more accurate figure, multiply your weight in kilos by 14.8 and add on 487. (This is a formula devised by the nutrition profession to calculate your calorie intake.)

For example, I weigh 57 kilos, which multiplied by 14.8 comes to 844. So 844 + 487 = 1331. This means I need a base rate of 1331 calories a day.

Most of us use about another 500 calories a day on top of the base rate for just mooching around, running for a bus, cleaning the house, etc., so bear that in mind when calculating your own.

When I feel I am becoming a little heavy and want to **reduce** my weight, I aim to eat around 1300 calories a day and increase my exercise routine. This will (hopefully) give me a weight loss of slightly under 1 kg a week, once my body has kicked into action, because like many people who try to cut down on their intake, I find that it seems to take about a week to ten days before I start to feel that the weight is slowly beginning to go down.

If, however, I wanted to **maintain** my weight, I would need to add those 500 calories to my 1331, making a total of 1800.

The heavier you are, the more calories you need each day just to tick over. But as you lose weight, so your basal metabolic rate needs to be adjusted downwards.

THE SIRENS OF WEIGHT GAIN

These are **fats** and **alcohol**. (I call them sirens because they are pleasurable whilst luring you into a false sense of well-being.) An excess of both are the main cause of weight gain, because gram for gram they have more calories than other foods.

One gram of fat contains 9 calories, and **one gram of alcohol contains 7 calories**, compared to one gram of carbo-hydrate or protein at 4 calories each.

Nutritionists advise that just over half of our daily intake of calories should come from carbohydrates and just over a third from fats. In fact, for many of us in the Western world, it is esti-mated that around 45% of our calories come from fat, which is a quarter too much.

In addition, we must also watch the **type** of fat. Harmful satu-rated fats are the ones that can cause health problems and the chief source of these are animal fats, which we should limit to around a tenth of our total fat intake.

We are all advised to cut our average fat intakes by a third. If you want to lose weight, you will need to cut this figure by a third again.

Recommended daily calorie and fat intakes			
Adult women	2000 calories	Fat intake	77g
Adult men	2500 calories	Fat intake	99g

From a health point of view, vegetarians score an advantage where fat is concerned because most vegetable fats are monounsaturated or polyunsaturated. But these healthier fats are still 9 calories per gram. However, some of the foods that non-meat eaters enjoy contain saturated fats from an animal source. These fats come in many forms and disguises; in dairy foods such as butter, cheese, cream and eggs, for example, but they are also to be found in chips, pastries, biscuits, ice cream and snacks. They all contain saturated fat. To complicate matters further, some saturated fats are of plant origin, such as coconut and palm oil.

It is helpful to understand this when trying to regulate the foods you consume. I have known overweight vegetarians who seem blissfully unaware that they are eating a high-fat diet. The basic principles of weight loss and weight maintenance are the same for *all* of us, carnivores, omnivores, vegetarians and even (albeit rarely) vegans.

If your calorie intake is the same as your energy output, you have one happy, bouncy, lean bunny. If it is more, you start to become one cuddly bigger bunny. So if your equation is tipping on the overweight side, you can either increase your energy output through exercise (see page 32) or decrease your calorie intake by watching the type and amount of food you eat (see Know What You Eat, Chapter 3, from page 37).

CHAPTER TWO

The Feel-Good Factor

MOTIVATION

Motivation is the first step to trimming weight, shape and size. Many diets fail because the root causes of the problem were not tackled in the first place. Before you look for a magic-wand solution, you should spend time looking in the mirror and asking yourself a few fundamental questions.

Physical factors such as hormone imbalance are rarely the cause of serious weight gain. But body type is inherited and has to be taken into consideration, so it is no good trying to look like a catwalk model if you don't have the basic structure for it. Be realistic. Aim to be as fit and healthy as you can, rather than an unnatural shape. Life is only unfair if that's the way you see it. Besides, fashions change. Being lean and lanky may be the media's current idea of perfect physiques, but we are all born with different attributes and talents, which we should strive to perfect. Just take advantage of your advantages.

ASK YOURSELF SOME FUNDAMENTAL QUESTIONS

Do you really want to lose weight and change your lifestyle or are you giving in to peer pressure? What factors were responsible for you putting on weight in the first place? Tackle the root cause before you handle the symptoms. Make a list of the bad aspects in your life.

For example, have you become overweight because you are badly depressed? If so, counselling or reading self-help books (borrow them free from a local library) may be a good long-term solution before you start to embark on a weight reducing diet. There are a number of weight reducing self-help groups with fantastic back-up support, like group therapy. Again, the local library or the phone directory will have contact numbers.

Do you overeat because you are bored? Are you isolated with few friends, little money and no transport? Have you just had a baby and the weight isn't shedding despite reassuring remarks by your health visitor?

These need not be excuses, merely factors that can be taken into account. Sadly, a vicious circle can be perpetuated: you eat because you are depressed about being overweight and lethargic.

How do you see yourself?
It is sometimes said that being seriously overweight is a form of hiding oneself away. Even when they have maybe only a stone or so to lose, some women will stop looking at their reflection in the mirror or when passing a shop window, afraid of what they might see. They cut down on going to the hairdresser as regularly, buy unshaped larger-size clothes and spend less time 'getting ready' in the morning. They even become introspective and stop chatting to friends. But when the weight starts to drop off, it's amazing how their self-confidence returns.

So, if you find your clothes getting a little tight, resist the temptation to buy the next size up. Keep wearing the same pair of jeans or waisted dress until you can breathe in it more comfortably because you have lost some weight.

THE DANGER OF DIETING

Twiggy, the first of the swinging sixties supermodels, unwittingly (bless her) spawned a whole new culture. Clothes moved rhythmically on her naturally lean and lithe frame and within weeks of her becoming the face of the decade, young women wanted to emulate her elfin, waif-like, vulnerable look. Gone was the desire to copy the curvy Marilyn Monroe. Bosoms were out and straight slim hips were in. Which was all very well, but only a very small percentage of women had the frame or metabolism for such a look.

With the swinging sixties came blue jeans, skimpy bikinis, miniskirts and hot pants. We had just emerged from the plain cooking decade of post-war rationing with plates piled high at mealtimes. People were becoming more aware of so-called exotic foods like peppers and aubergines. Magazines started running articles on miracle diets that could turn you into a lean, cool chick: 'Lose pounds in a week' screamed their front-cover headlines. Diet gurus began to

> *There is still this notion that to slim, one must follow a formula diet and suffer from hunger, and that once the goal of lean and trim is reached, one can magically return to the former way of eating ...*

appear, telling us that eating bread and potatoes made you fat, yet lots of high-protein steak or cheese made you lean. Miracle cures were offered by extraordinary diets, such as peanuts and oranges, or grapefruit and crispbread for breakfast, lunch and supper – all based on the notion that if you went on a 'crash diet' for a fortnight or more, your body would benefit and the slim inner you would emerge, ready to take the world by storm.

What is quite extraordinary about such dated notions is that some of them continue to survive some forty years on, not only in the psyche of those of us around in the sixties and seventies, but regrettably in those of a whole generation who have grown up subsequently. There is still this notion that to slim, one must follow a formula diet and suffer from hunger, and that once the goal of lean and trim is reached, one can magically return to the former way of eating. We were led to believe that the secret of successful slimming relied on miracle diets with endless lists and plans (a theory that seems to linger on in the minds of some diet gurus and publishers). Sadly this short, sharp, shock treatment has little long-term

> *... sadly this short, sharp, shock treatment has little long-term effect.*

> *It is better to have one long diet of a few months with effects that last a lifetime.*

effect and a great number of 'dieters' seem to reoffend, often becoming more overweight than before. Why?

The human race evolved and was able to disperse through continents with a great variety of climates by being adaptable. When our hunter-gatherer ancestors fell on lean times, their bodies were able to adjust by absorbing surplus energy laid down in times of plenty in the form of body fat – but if lean times turned into famine, the body started to absorb its own lean tissue to supply it with energy just to stay alive. Similarly, thousand of years on, if we diet for too long and deprive ourselves of energy and nutrients, our bodies go into starvation mode, our basal metabolic rate plummets and we start to absorb good lean tissue. Then when we start to eat normally again, and the weight starts to creep back up, instead of restoring that lean tissue, we store what is now *excess* energy as fat tissue. Hence the term 'yo-yo' diet and the maxim 'Dieting can make you fat'.

What is needed is not crash formula diets for instant results but a long, steady re-education of our eating habits so that when we lose weight, we lose the right sort of weight (i.e. body fat), which stays off for ever. It is better to have one long diet of a few months with effects that last a lifetime than to start several, each lasting a couple of weeks, which all fail and make you more miserable than ever.

So, what's so great about sensible eating?

Before you even start to think about 'dieting' take time to learn about a healthy diet – what you actually eat. It sounds like a cliché, but think of your body like a car. You only fill it with a certain grade of fuel, use the right type of oil, top up with battery water, put low-lather screenwash in the windscreen washer pouch and take it to the garage for regular servicing. In return you get years of trouble-free motoring. In the same way, our bodies need particular nutrients for all our complicated functions to run smoothly. And just as many of us don't know what goes on under the bonnet of a car, so it is a little alarming that our knowledge of our own dietary needs is so inaccurate. The human body is not only more sophisticated than a car, it is truly amazing!

BASIC HEALTHY EATING

With all the apparently conflicting advice about what foods we should and shouldn't eat, it's not surprising that most of us get very confused, even without all the so-called miracle or theme diets that have hit the headlines.

In my youth, starchy foods were seen as the baddies, and to lose weight we were told to stick to salads and high-protein foods. But this was a misinterpretation of the facts; it was not starchy or carbohydrate foods that were causing the weight gain, but the amount of fat we seemed to eat with them. In other words, it was not the bread that had the high calories but the butter spread lavishly over it; not the potatoes that were cut into chips but the oil they were deep-fried in; not the pasta but the rich creamy sauce with cheese on top.

Now we are advised to include good amounts of bread, potatoes, pasta and rice in our meals, lots of fresh vegetables and fruit, with only moderate amounts of protein, modest amounts of 'good' fats and small amounts of sugar.

To help us understand this easily and clear up any confusion, nutritionists advise that over half our calories should come from **carbohydrates**: cereals, grains, potatoes, rice and pasta.

We should include as much **fresh fruit and vegetables** as we can manage – ideally, at least five good portions a day, even if one of them is just a glass of fresh orange juice.

We need surprisingly little **protein**, taken from pulses, eggs, dairy foods, nuts, cheese and seeds.

Finally, **fats, oils and sugary foods** should be taken in small amounts.

But remember: the principle still holds good when you eat these foods together. So if you have a slice of bread, spread the butter very thinly; choose a low-sugar or sugar-free cereal; boil or poach eggs rather than fry them in a lot of oil, and so on.

> **The main message, however, for all lean eating is variety and balance. If you eat a lot of different types of food from the main nutrition food groups – carbohydrates, proteins, fats, vitamins and minerals – there is little for you to worry about. You can forget the fancy formulas, as long as you don't OD on fats and empty sugary foods.**

Let's look at these food groups in more detail.

THE FOOD PYRAMID

To simplify matters, nutritionists advise us to think of our diet as a 3-D pyramid divided into sections.

At the base (more than half of the total area) are **starchy complex carbohydrate foods** – ironically all the foods that we were advised to cut down on thirty years ago. Nutritionists divide carbohydrates into two types – simple and complex. Both give us energy, but simple carbohydrates, namely sugars, give us a quick fix of energy, nothing more. They are quickly absorbed and quickly used up. Complex carbohydrates are absorbed more slowly and steadily into the bloodstream, in what is known as slow-release energy, and so in terms of calories given, they are better value. This is why athletes like to 'carbo load' before a big race to store up slow-release energy to keep them going for longer. Carbohydrates should make up 55% of your diet, or six servings a day.

Well, now that it's official, let's shout it out – BREAD, PASTA, RICE, POTATOES, CEREALS AND GRAINS ARE GOOD FOR YOU!

The next main group are **vegetables and fruit.** In the main, these do not give us great amounts of energy (calories) but they do contain vital vitamins and minerals, which are necessary to enable certain body functions to take place (see Full of Vim and Vit, page 58).

For example, vitamins of the B group are needed for our bodies to absorb the energy from carbohydrates; vitamin C assists the absorption of iron (especially from vegetable sources); vitamin D works in tandem with calcium, and so on. They also look good, taste delicious and we

> *Vegetables and fruit look good, taste delicious and we can eat them as freely as we please.*

can eat them as freely as we please, with a minimum suggested allowance of five portions a day (see Five a Day, page 44).

Going further up the pyramid are **protein and dairy foods**. Choose two to three small servings of each per day. Proteins are vital for the proper functioning of all our body cells. We do need

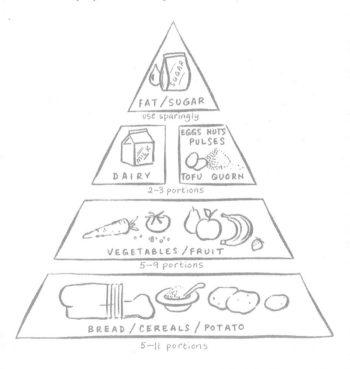

FAT / SUGAR
use sparingly

DAIRY   EGGS NUTS PULSES
               TOFU QUORN
2-3 portions

VEGETABLES / FRUIT
5-9 portions

BREAD / CEREALS / POTATO
5-11 portions

a sufficient supply in a normal balanced diet, whether slimming or maintaining our weight.

But, it may surprise you to learn that we don't actually need great amounts of protein once we've emerged from our teens and stopped growing. After that, we need just a small amount of protein for cell repair. The Recommended Daily Amounts (RDAs) are around 45g for adult women, and 55g for men. Anything eaten over and above that figure is used up either as energy or stored as body fat. Yet somehow the myth persists in the current fad for low-carbo diets that you need to cut down on starchy foods and eats lots of 'lean' protein.

Vegetarians have a great advantage over meat eaters, as long as they are aware of the basic facts concerning proteins. Vegetable protein foods are lower in fat.

Proteins are a mixture of organic compounds contained as molecules made up of chains of amino acids, like building blocks. Our bodies need nine essential amino acids for all the various functions to keep us healthy. Flesh foods (meat and fish) contain all these amino acids but in the case of meat these proteins can come with the additional liability of saturated fats. There are many vegetable and flesh-free sources of proteins too although they may not contain the complete complement of essential amino acids. But this should present no problem because vegetable proteins (without saturated fats) come in a naturally occurring variety pack – you simply mix and match.

The best rule of thumb to ensure a good supply of essential amino acids is to eat grains and pulses or nuts or eggs in the same meal. So, the amino acids missing from say, beans may be present in wheat or potatoes or rice. Over the centuries, man has instinctively sussed this out and many cultures eat combinations of grains and pulses – lentils and rice, tofu and noodles, hummus and pitta, rice and peas, baked beans on toast.

Dairy products (and eggs) are excellent sources of proteins – milk, cheese, yogurts, fromage frais, etc., but as these can be high in animal saturated fats, try to eat lower- or reduced-fat versions instead. (See page 48 on lower-fat dairy foods.)

Dairy foods (including lower-fat versions) are good sources of minerals such as calcium, magnesium and selenium, plus vitamins B1, B2 and B12. Egg yolks contain vitamins A, B1, B2 and D, plus the minerals iron and zinc. However, they also contain a form of cholesterol, so if you already have a blood cholesterol problem, you should be aware of this. Those without such a problem can actually eat an egg a day – good news for healthy vegetarians.

At the very tip of our healthy eating pyramid, to be eaten in cautious amounts, are **fats and sugars.** Fats have over double the calories per gram of proteins and carbohydrates but they are also rich sources of certain vital vitamins – A, D, E and K – so don't exclude them completely. These vitamins are just as abundant in lower-fat products and can be found in non-fat foods such as green leafy vegetables, pulses, eggs and whole grains.

A little dollop of half-fat crème fraiche, a teaspoon or two of olive or sunflower or soya oil, a light spreading of polyunsaturated margarine, even a knob of butter or small scoop of ice cream are fine, indeed vital, for our general health. Fats and sugars give us a nice sense of well-being – but we should leave it at that. Treat them as treats. Fats should account for no more than a third of our daily calorie intake, and sugars just a tenth.

CALORIE COUNTING

Recommended daily calories
Adult women 2000
Adult men 2500
(See also Body Mass Index and basal metabolic rate, page 15.)

Whether you are losing weight or trying to maintain the new slimmer you, it is useful to have a good idea of the calorie values of foods so that you don't slip back into the old ways. (See Appendix, page 140, for a list of the most common calorie figures.)

Remember, adult women are advised to keep within an

approximate figure of 2000 calories a day, 2500 for adult men, to **maintain** their current weight. On average, these figures should decrease by a quarter to **reduce** weight.

For healthy eating, keep an eye on **fat** figures too.

Daily fat levels
Normal fat levels – Adult men should aim for no more than 99g fat per day; adult women 77g fat per day.
To lose weight – Reduce your fat levels to at least 85g a day for men and 67g for women.

Some slimming organizations work on a points system, which is fine, but if you are not following their particular method you might feel a bit uncertain about what to eat when you return to normal or if you are away from home. Also, for many people who live on their own, cooking specific recipes is not always practical (however desirable), yet they still want to eat well. However, if you know the approximate calorie and fat values of foods, then you know when you can treat yourself without tripping up. Forewarned is forearmed. It also helps you develop a more balanced approach to healthy eating.

READING NUTRITION LABELS

One of the best sources of information about the food you eat is the nutrition boxes printed on product labels. Slowly, more companies are divulging information about the calorie, fat, carbohydrate, fibre, salt and vitamin levels in their foods. This helps you make an informed choice.

At the moment supermarkets (and breakfast cereal manufacturers) lead the way in user-friendly labelling that is easy to read; often figures are given in useful portion sizes. Some manufacturers give all their products a common denominator, so that you can compare like with like, and they provide figures per 100g or 100ml of product. Although this may often bear no relation to the amounts in which you eat foods, it still gives you a working framework. Take time to familiarize yourself with these labels and gradually you will be able to quickly ascertain whether foods are suitable for your balanced eating regime or better kept as occasional treats.

You may also find some labels give percentages of **RDAs** of certain vitamins, fibre, etc. This refers to the **Recommended Dietary Allowances** for nutrients, set by government guidelines. Please don't feel you must follow them slavishly, life is too short, but it will give you an idea of which foods are good sources of say, fibre or a certain B group vitamin, so that you can think within broad outlines. However, the best advice for keeping within the RDAs for vitamins and minerals is to eat five good portions of fruit and vegetables a day (see page 44). Follow this and there's no need to worry about exact figures.

Fibre facts

Fibre figures are important too, not just for weight control but for healthy lifestyles. In itself, fibre has no calories but it is essential to help carry waste products effortlessly through our digestive system so that they can be excreted without strain on our intestines.

Fibre (derived from plant fibres) is divided into two types: insoluble and soluble. A good intake of **insoluble fibre**, found in whole grains, bran and vegetable skins, helps to fill you up and make you feel less hungry. Such fibre swells up with water and carries waste products along with it as it passes through the gut. It cannot be absorbed through the gut walls and so remains intact. Soft waste products put less pressure on the gut as they pass through and so help prevent diseases such as colon cancer.

Soluble fibre, found in many plant foods but particularly in oats, barley, rye and beans, does pass through the gut wall and is absorbed into the bloodstream. It acts as a type of scouring agent, cleaning cholesterol from the blood and thus reducing the risk of high blood pressure and ultimately heart attack.

> *Insoluble fibre helps your digestion and 'fills' you up without calories.*

To recap, insoluble fibre helps your digestion and 'fills' you up without calories, so it is ideal when you want to reduce your calorie intake. Soluble fibre is good for your general health. Bear these points in mind when you read food labels.

We are advised to eat 27 to 40 grams of fibre a day. Don't OD on fibre, however, as bran contains substances known as phytates, which can inhibit the absorption of certain minerals. As a general principle, just try to eat a third more high-fibre foods each day and change from white starchy foods to brown where possible.

High-fibre foods include all wholegrain foods (generally brown or wholemeal versions of starchy foods), vegetables and pulses with skins.

WHAT ARE YOU DRINKING?

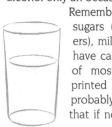

As a general rule, you should try to drink around 2 litres of liquid a day, much of it in the form of plain water. Bottled mineral or straight from the tap, it doesn't matter. Some of this can be in the form of tea or coffee.

Carbonated drinks, fruit juices and non-alcoholic cordials should be in addition, and alcohol only an occasional treat.

Remember: if a drink contains sugars (not artificial sweeteners), milk or alcohol it will also have calories. The calorie level of most soft drinks will be printed on the label so it is probably a safe bet to assume that if no figures are given, the item is quite high in calories (see page 144).

ALCOHOL

First the bad news. Pure alcohol contains 7 calories per gram, although if an alcoholic drink is diluted with sugary mixers or cream, the calories increase. It is quickly absorbed into the

> A glass or two of red wine in the evening, with food, can be part of a normal healthy lifestyle. But do your liver a favour and have at least two alcohol-free days a week.

system, especially on an empty stomach, and is slowly broken down by the liver, so the after-effects remain for some time. Also alcohol acts as a diuretic so it will dehydrate you more quickly.

In addition it is recommended that you drink no more than the equivalent of 1 unit of alcohol per hour to limit potential damage to the liver. The calories from alcohol that are not used as energy are stored as body fat. Alcohol that is reduced down in cooking counts as zero units.

Medical professionals measure alcohol in units. A normal glass of wine will contain 1.5 units, a half-pint of light lager or beer 1 unit, and a small shot of spirits 1 unit.

For safe drinking levels, women are advised to follow a guideline of a maximum of 21 units a week, 28 units a week for men, but it is not recommended that you store up your units for a once-weekly binge. Think of your liver, please!

And now, a wee dram of good news. Moderate drinking of alcohol in association with food by normal healthy people will do little harm. It helps us to relax and contributes to stress relief, hence combating what is thought to be one of the main causes of heart and blood pressure problems. Indeed, red wine is thought to have some medical benefit by keeping blood platelets flowing freely. A glass or two of red wine in the evening, with food, can be part of a normal healthy lifestyle.

But do your liver a favour and have at least two alcohol-free days a week – it needs time off. If you are following a weight reducing diet, allow for the fact that a small glass (125ml) of wine can have 85 calories and a small lite beer 120 calories, so it makes sense to use your calorie allowance more sensibly than taking in empty calories.

EXERCISE

Changing your diet or planning long-term weight maintenance can only really be effective if you kick-start your metabolic rate into a higher gear and that means incorporating meaningful exercise into your new regime. You will also find that after a while, exercise will lift your spirits and make you feel better. Our brains secrete natural painkilling chemicals called endorphins, which make you feel really good after physical exercise, a condition sometimes called 'runner's high'. It doesn't happen immediately but as you get into a routine of regular exercise, you should find that you begin to feel better, and conversely if you cannot do your regular routine for whatever reason, you may become grumpy!

Start slowly and take your time to build up a routine. No one is so busy that they can't slot 20 minutes into each day of some form of aerobic activity. It doesn't have to be an organized sport that needs planning ahead. Even gardening can keep you fit. One effective form of exercise is walking, at a brisk speed somewhere between strolling and almost running when your arms automatically rise into a half-folded position.

If you really are emerging from couch potato status, or have never exercised seriously before, this is the best way to start even if it takes you a couple of months or so to progress on to another energy level. Just change aspects of your daily life gradually. Instead of taking a lift or escalators, take the stairs or at least a couple of flights. Walk to the station instead of waiting for a bus or, even worse, driving! If the station is too far away, cycle. If you are home-based, instead of sitting down after a light lunch to watch a soap, go for a walk (and video the soap!)

Exercise will lift your spirits and make you feel better.

Soon exercise will be part of your daily lifestyle and you'll begin to feel you have new energy levels, which make you want to do more. Then you can consider an additional form of exercise. From walking you may progress to gentle jogging, alternating the two in the same period. That is, walk briskly for 10 minutes, then break into a jog for 5 minutes, go back to walking

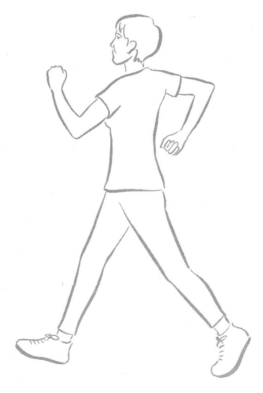

> *Set yourself little exercise goals each day or change them each week.*

and so on. Very soon the jogging time in between gets longer. Set yourself little exercise goals each day or change them each week. Increase the number of laps round the park or add another street to your route.

Exercise for weight maintenance can be divided into two forms: **aerobic exercise**, which works the heart and lungs and helps burn calories, and **stretch conditioning**, which tones and reshapes your muscles.

Aerobic exercise is categorized by intensity levels – low, medium and high, depending on the amount of respiration and breathlessness you reach. Aerobic exercise also raises your basal metabolic rate (see page 15), which increases the number of calories you burn up when just resting. Double bonus, really.

Other good examples of aerobic exercises that build up stamina are **jogging** (gentle, progressing to trotting speed), **swimming**, **cycling** and **dancing**.

If you are a winter sports fan, **cross-country skiing** is a brilliant alternative to flying down the piste.

Aerobic dancing is a great fun way of not only enjoying funky music played at full blast but also of meeting other people, an important move if you feel isolated. You don't have to get the latest in chic designer gear. Leggings and a baggy T-shirt are absolutely fine. That's what most of us start out wearing.

Tennis is also not only excellent exercise but one of the best ways of meeting people and making new social contacts, especially useful if one of the reasons for your change in lifestyle is that you want to break out of loneliness.

Swimming is regarded as the best all-round exercise as your weight is supported by the water and the impact on joints is minimized. This assumes, of course, that you have a good pool within travelling distance, which has special areas dedicated to lane swimming. Again, start slowly, resting after every two or three lengths, and gradually build up speed over the months.

Try to do 20–30 minutes of some form of aerobic exercise four times a week plus two stretch and conditioning sessions too. In addition to burning calories and increasing the efficiency of your heart rate with aerobic exercise, you also need to keep your muscles supple and toned.

Examples of stretch classes are yoga, Pilates, jazz ballet and, my favourite, Lotte Berk, on which the American Callanetics is based.

If you don't have suitable classes near you there are numerous stretch techniques on video, which will last and last until the tape wears out!

How many calories do you burn per hour?
- Basal metabolism (e.g. sleeping) – 65 calories
- Walking – 250 calories
- Cycling, medium pace – 300 calories
- Jogging – 400 calories
- Swimming, medium pace – 500 calories
- Squash – 650 calories

The benefits of regular exercise
- Protects against disease such as cancers, heart attacks, high blood pressure
- Tones and strengthens muscles
- Uses up calories
- Strengthens bones
- Benefits your lungs and increases oxygen uptake
- Improves blood circulation
- Keeps your body flexible and your joints mobile
- Makes you feel happy
- Helps you sleep and feel less anxious

So, what are you waiting for?

CHAPTER THREE

Know What You Eat

CARBOHYDRATES
BREAD

Few of us can imagine a daily diet without bread. It appears at nearly every meal. Toast for breakfast, sandwiches for lunch, rolls at dinner – and in between more toast for snacks. Not to mention the terrific variety of ethnic and fat enriched 'fancy' breads such as croissants, brioche and, dare I mention, doughnuts?

Basic bread contains complex carbohydrate (from 41g per 100g for wholemeal to 49g for white) plus protein, dietary fibre, vitamins of the B group, added iron and calcium and just a very small amount of fat. All for around 80–83 calories per medium slice. It is a very good source of energy so don't cut it out.

Officially, we are recommended to eat the equivalent of 6 slices of bread a day, but this assumes you don't eat many other complex carbohydrates. Certainly, a couple of slices of morning toast and maybe a roll for lunch can be easily included each day. Like other complex carbos, bread is also a good source of fibre – better than fruit and vegetables. And, remember it is the fat we spread on bread that increases the calories.

> **Bread is a good source of fibre – better than fruit and vegetables.**

Grainy breads give us extra fibre as well as flavour. Rye breads give a tangy, slightly acidic flavour and moist chewy texture but most rye bread sold in the UK is mixed with wheat flour, so if you have a wheat allergy check the labels first. There are a few all-rye breads like Borodinsky and pumpernickel.

Wheat Grains

Bread is made from the ground flour of wheat grains, but the grains themselves can be eaten in other healthy forms. The best known is couscous – tiny ground grains of wheat semolina which needs to be soaked then briefly steamed (or microwaved) and served hot with spicy stews or tossed with vinaigrette for salads. Really easy to prepare and cook, although I would recommend you fork the soaked grains well to separate them before serving. Bulghur wheat (aka cracked wheat and pourgouri) are parboiled wheat grains which simply need soaking. Brilliant for salads like the classic Tabbouleh (see recipe page 80) mixed lightly with a trickle of olive oil, fresh lemon juice and lots of fresh green herbs. Spelt is an ancient form of wheat grain (aka Farro) popular with Roman soldiers as they marched around conquering great tracts of Europe in the 1st century AD.

POTATOES

The humble spud once had an illustrious past. Ladies of the glamorous 18th century French court would wear the dainty flowers in their hair, but it wasn't until the efforts of a French chemist Parmentier that it was realized what a highly nutritious food the potato was. Like bread, rice and pasta, potatoes are a good source of complex carbohydrates full of energy and, if the skins are included, high in fibre, with virtually no fat unless you dollop it with butter or soured cream. But potatoes are also fresh vegetables so full of vitamins C, B6 and potassium. New potatoes are the highest in vitamin C, especially if freshly harvested. Baked jacket potatoes are wonderful for increasing your fibre intake, but deep fried chips will increase calories by up to 3 times. You must decide if it is worth it. A 200g microwaved baked potato at a modest 144 calories is one of the best low fat, high carbohydrate healthy meals you can have, especially teamed with a small can of baked beans.

> *New potatoes are the highest in vitamin C, especially if freshly harvested.*

PASTAS

As a complex carbohydrate food and therefore high in starch, pasta is a valuable part of a healthy diet whether you are following a weight-reducing or a weight-maintenance plan. In itself, pasta does not make you fat, as long as you eat a normal-size portion with the smallest possible amount of accompanying oil or fats such as butter or cream, or better still a fat-free sauce.

In itself, pasta does not make you fat.

Pastas are sold dried or 'fresh'; that is, still pliable rather than brittle, but as this type can come vacuum-packed it is debatable how fresh is fresh. In Italy, real fresh pasta is only made in homes or restaurants. Most Italians use dried pastas, made from hard durum wheat semolina and water. Egg pastas are richer. There are also various coloured pastas, which contain spinach, beetroot, tomatoes or even squid ink.

A 100g quantity of dried pasta will provide around 360 calories, which is a very generous portion. You should generally reckon on about 75g uncooked weight per person, which when it is cooked and bulked up with water comes out at around 270 calories. It is still good, lean and light food for the base of a main meal. Serve with a fresh tomato sauce, such as in the recipe below, rather than dripping with oil, butter or rich sauces such as pesto, mascarpone or four-cheese.

Always buy the best-quality branded pasta you can afford – there is quite a difference between brands. And check for the words 100% durum wheat pasta on the packs.

Those with a wheat allergy might like to look out for rice flour or corn pastas – they actually make reasonable substitutes, albeit with different textures.

FRESH TOMATO SAUCE

This is a good recipe for a light, quick pasta sauce. The alcohol is not essential, but is very flavoursome. Top the sauce with a sprinkling of grated fresh parmesan or lashings of freshly grated nutmeg.

Makes enough for 150g (dried weight) pasta
Serves 2
Calories per portion/serving: 60

INGREDIENTS
4 ripe plum tomatoes
1 small onion, chopped
2 teaspoons olive oil
2 fat cloves garlic, crushed
2 tablespoons dry vermouth or white wine (optional)
sea salt and freshly ground black pepper

METHOD
Peel the tomatoes by dipping them briefly in boiling water, then stripping off the skins. Cut in quarters, remove the core and chop roughly, including the seeds.

Sauté the onion in the oil and 2 tablespoons water for about 5 minutes. Add the garlic, the chopped tomatoes and the dry vermouth or white wine, if using.

Simmer uncovered for 5 minutes, stirring occasionally until pulpy. Season well. Mix in either 1–2 good pinches of dried oregano or 1–2 tablespoons chopped fresh basil. Serve.

Choosing and cooking pasta
Long thin skinny pasta shapes suit light sauces that coat but don't cling. Pasta shapes with hollows or tubes trap pools of sauce inside and so suit thicker, juicy or creamier sauces.

Boil pasta in plenty of lightly salted boiling water. A really good pasta will not go soggy even if slightly overcooked and it will never stick to itself during cooking. Italians always serve their pastas slightly wet; in other words they don't shake them dry after boiling and draining. It's a useful tip for those watching calories, so you don't have to smother pasta in sauce to keep it moist. Good ole water is ideal.

Wholewheat pasta is higher in fibre and slightly lower in calories but you may find the texture slightly chewy. Personally, I like it – it's particularly good with ratatouille and chickpeas.

ORIENTAL NOODLES

Without getting into the debate about whether it was the Italians or the Chinese who 'invented' pasta, you can ring the changes in your diet by eating Chinese, Japanese or Thai noodles made of wheat and other grains, namely rice, buckwheat and the supergrain, quinoa. Cook them in the same way as pasta, but serve them either simply dressed with soy sauce or miso or with a bowl of steamed vegetables. Very thin rice noodles need just soaking in boiling water for 15–20 minutes.

Noodles made with other grains tend to be a bit on the chewy side but once you get used to them they are an invaluable ingredient and highly nutritious. Particularly tasty are Japanese Udon noodles made of buckwheat. Although they are a somewhat unprepossessing brown colour, they have a delicious flavour. I enjoy them in clear soups or miso broths as a light lunch or snack.

RICE

Another good high-starch complex carbohydrate food, rice is great at filling you up with lots of energy and little or no fat. A 100g quantity, uncooked weight, will give you around 350 calories, about the same as pasta, enough for one and a half portions. Rice is also a valuable source of B group vitamins and minerals such as selenium and zinc – all good at keeping you bright-eyed and bushy-tailed.

Although rice lacks the Mediterranean glamour of pasta, it is in fact a far more versatile all-round food. Not for nothing is rice

> *Rice is great at filling you up with lots of energy and little or no fat and is also a valuable source of B group vitamins and minerals.*

the staple crop of over half the world's population. In China, for instance, they eat nearly 80 kilos per head per annum – breakfast, lunch and dinner.

Rice is very digestible and is one of the cleansing foods recommended for 'detox' diets. The aromatic or fragrant rices are the nicest – basmati and Thai jasmine. They take just 10 minutes to cook and need very little else in the way of additional flavourings. Again, choose good branded rices as their quality is consistent.

Rice is a grain that has simply been dehusked and refined lightly, not made into a paste like pasta, so the original grain is more important.

The amount and type of starch in the rice determines the texture of the cooked rice dish. Risotto rices have higher levels of starch, which when stirred during cooking comes out into the dish and makes it taste creamy without high fat. Then you can add whatever flavourings and extra ingredients you like. Most people adore a bowl of real risotto – almost the ultimate comfort food – but it does need to be made properly and eaten immediately. Follow the recipe on page 116.

Rinsing and soaking rice

It is not necessary to rinse and soak rice if you are using good branded types, as they are all cleaned anyway, but it does help to lighten the grain if you want a more authentic rice for curries, especially high-quality basmati.

To rinse rice – tip whatever quantity you want (I would recommend not less than 100g at a time) into a big bowl and fill with cold running water. Swirl the grains with your hand, count to three, then tip out the water. The wet grains will sink to the bottom. Fill with water again and repeat the swirling and draining. On the fourth or fifth rinse, leave the rice in the water and soak for 15–20 minutes. Then drain in a colander. After this you will need to shorten the cooking time by as much as half. Check the pack label for details.

Cooking rice

If you have any problems cooking rice, follow either of these two simple methods.

Method 1: Open-pan boiling Treat rice as you would pasta: boil it in lots of lightly salted boiling water. Bring a large pan of water to the boil, tip in the rice, stir once or twice and return to a medium boil. Cook uncovered for the following times:
- basmati and Thai – 10 minutes (6–7 minutes if soaked).
- American long grain and easy-cook – 15–20 minutes
- brown – 20–40 minutes (brown basmati is the quickest-cooking and the best for flavour and fibre)
- wild – 45–50 minutes (or soak overnight and cook for 20 minutes)

Method 2: Absorption/covered pan This method is easy to follow but not as good for light fluffy grains. It is suitable for easy-cook, basmati, brown, wild and Thai rices. Simply measure your chosen rice in a jug or cup and add water in the following proportions:
- basmati and Thai – $1\frac{1}{2}$ cups water to 1 cup rice
- American long grain and easy-cook – 2 cups water to 1 cup rice
- brown and Carmargue red rice – $2–2\frac{1}{2}$ cups water to 1 cup rice
- wild – $2\frac{1}{2}$ cups water to 1 cup rice

Bring to the boil, stir once, turn the heat right down, cover and cook (see cooking times below, measured from when the water returns to the boil). No peeking or lifting the lid or you will let out precious steam and moisture.
- basmati and Thai – 10 minutes
- American long grain and easy-cook – 15–20 minutes
- brown basmati and Carmargue red rice – 25 minutes
- brown – 40 minutes
- wild – 45–50 minutes

At the end of the cooking time, remove the pan from the heat, still covered, then fork through the grains.

FRUIT AND VEGETABLES
EAT FIVE A DAY

You can forget all the minutiae of what vitamins and minerals to eat each day simply by thinking in terms of eating five modest portions each of fresh fruit and vegetables, as long as they are a mixed selection. It's the variety that is important. Vegetarians are bound to eat more fresh vegetables and fruit because they tend to have a more interesting and varied diet. So, if there is to be a formula in your diet, let it be this simple one.

Eat Five a Day
'Fresh, frozen, cooked or raw – it doesn't really matter, just eat more!'

Putting it into practice

It is in fact very easy to 'eat five a day'. The actual amounts involved are quite small. Nor does it have to be fresh produce. You can include fresh fruit juices (not squash or fruit drinks), frozen vegetables and even the juice of a lemon in a dressing.

Potatoes, however, are not included, as they count as carbo-hydrates.

Also, you only need aim for modest portions of around 80g a time, which is the prepared weight – a minimum total of 400g. As most fruits and vegetables come in sizes larger than that, it soon becomes easy to reach this target. A small apple, banana or pear weigh around 100g each, a medium tomato is 80g, 2 small carrots are 100g, 3 tablespoons peas, a very small glass of fresh orange juice, 1 little gem lettuce, a small courgette and so on are around 100g/100ml.

Eat five modest portions each of fresh fruit and vegetables, as long as they are a mixed selection.

A typical example of **Five a Day** would be: a glass of fresh orange juice and 1 banana for breakfast, 1 sliced tomato in a lunchtime sandwich, 1/2 onion, 2 carrots and maybe some peas for the evening meal.

In fact that little amount adds up to 6 portions and most vegetarians eat more fresh produce than that a day. Or, put another way, just include one or two fresh items with each meal.

As we have already seen, fruit and vegetables are rich sources of vitamins and minerals. See Full of Vim and Vit, page 58, for more information.

You can also increase your intake by eating home-sprouted beans and seeds (see page 85).

PROTEINS AND DAIRY FOODS
PULSES

Pulses are the seeds of legumes. Beans are boat shaped, peas round. All are great sources of complex carbohydrates, fibre, vegetable proteins and minerals with calorie counts of around 140–160 per 100g uncooked weight. (To calculate the cooked value, dried pulses bulk out to about 2 1/2 times when cooked.) There are literally hundreds of varieties from quick cook split red lentils through to soya beans and chickpeas, which can take over an hour to cook. They are one of the great vegetarian mainstays – versatile, filling, healthy, easy to store in a cupboard and above all cheap. Make sure you include a pulse in one of your meals at least once a day, even if it is just a small can of baked beans.

NUTS

Nuts are rich in oils and are therefore high in calories but they are excellent sources of plant proteins and fibre, which as a vegetarian you will need – but just watch your intake.

> *Nuts are rich in oils and are therefore high in calories but they are excellent sources of plant proteins and fibre ... but just watch your intake.*

The nuts highest in fat are **brazils** (almost two-thirds fat) but they are also one of the best sources of the wonder mineral, selenium.

Next highest are **walnuts**, **peanuts** and **almonds** at half-fat, followed by **hazelnuts** and **white coconut flesh** at one-third fat.

Chestnuts are much lower in fat and have a good amount of starchy carbohydrate, so don't wait until Christmas time to eat them. Chinese stores sell packs of dried chestnuts, which when rehydrated taste as good as fresh. Italian delis often sell chestnut flour so if you want a reasonably lower-fat source of protein, include some in your cooking.

The richest nuts in terms of **protein** are peanuts, at around 25%, which makes them higher in protein than cheese.

In terms of calories you are looking at between 400 and 740 calories per 100g, depending on the nut. Brazils and pecans are the highest in calories, along with fresh cob nuts, at 400 calories per 100g. Chestnuts, however, are only 170 calories per 100g.

To make nuts go further, and taste more 'nutty' (so you use less), spread them in a shallow roasting pan and toast them in the oven at 180°C, Gas Mark 4, for around 12–15 minutes or until lightly golden brown. Then to make them go even further, chop them up to sprinkle over dishes. Make up a batch and store what you don't need in a screw-topped jar.

It is a good idea to work out the weight of nuts that you can eat in terms of calories for one meal and measure it in spoon sizes; then you know how much you can sprinkle over per meal in future without having to get out the scales each time.

SEEDS

Seeds are wonderful additions to the vegetarian store cupboard because they are high in minerals, but again, weight for weight, they are high in calories and fats.

The top of the list are **sesame seeds** – at around 640 calories per 100g – but then who would eat that many sesame seeds at once? A scant teaspoon (2g) at a time is fine. Even better, toast them lightly first to develop the flavour.

Treat **poppy seeds** and **linseeds** in the same way. **Sunflower** and **pumpkin seeds** are great in salads or scattered over vegetable casseroles.

TOFU

Although a non-dairy product, tofu is often sold in chilled cabinets alongside dairy products.

First developed over 800 years ago by Buddhists as a non-animal, high-protein food, it is a mainstay ingredient in many Chinese and Japanese dishes. I

> *A non-animal, high-protein food, tofu is a mainstay ingredient in many Chinese and Japanese dishes.*

love it but it is an acquired taste, or rather, as it has no taste in its natural state, it is a taste that you can grow to like simply because it takes on the flavour of other ingredients in the same dish, or can be cooked in such a way that it becomes tasty. It's the texture that you will have to get used to, rather like junket.

Very lean and low fat (around 90 calories per 100g), tofu is sold either as a light cream, called silken tofu (fabulous as a salad dressing or stirred in soup, as well as a good substitute for single cream), or pressed into semi-firm 'cakes' to be cut in cubes for adding to sauces, casseroles or stir-fries. For the best flavour choose marinated or smoked tofu. The Chinese and Japanese deep-fry cubes of tofu but as this increases the calories, I tend instead to grill a slab until the outside becomes crisp and then cut it into cubes, or dry-fry cubes in a hot non-stick pan sprayed first with some low-fat cooking spray.

SOYA

They may be dull to eat and take up to 2 hours to cook, but when processed soya beans are truly wonder foods. They can be made into milks (ideal for those with a dairy milk intolerance), tofu curds, fat spreads and textured vegetable proteins such as dried soya chunks or finer mince to be reconstituted with water and made into sauces, stews, burgers, etc. But take care when eating ready meals and vegetarian sausages or burgers with soya because they can also contain high amounts of fat, so check the pack label for fat percentages. Soya products are particularly good for women of menopause age because they contain good amounts of natural oestrogens.

QUORN

In the 1960s, scientists spent a lot of time and money looking for a very cheap, high-protein food to feed the Third World. One of the spin-offs of their research was the discovery of a myco-protein grown from a tiny fungus. This was developed into a product that is now sold under the brand name of Quorn and it is used increasingly in the production of vegetarian ready-meals.

Like tofu, it has no natural flavouring and takes on the taste of whatever it is cooked with. In addition to being high in a non-animal protein, and low in calories (around 55g per portion), it is very low in fat, cholesterol-free and a good source of fibre to boot! You can buy it in cubes or minced, and it takes just minutes to cook. The texture is a little artificial perhaps, but nevertheless, it is a good addition to a lean, healthy diet.

LOWER-FAT DAIRY FOODS

The last decade has seen a boom in the number of fat-reduced products appearing in chilled cabinets, dairy products particularly. This is good news as dairy products are excellent sources of proteins, vitamins and minerals, especially calcium.

Nutritional labelling has meant that we can now check on fat levels in food, which are usually expressed as grams per 100g of product. Sometimes this will be further subdivided into saturates, so you can keep a check on these too. The calorie content (expressed as **kcals**) will also give you a clue as to whether or not the food is suitable for a weight control diet.

Dairy products described as 'half-fat' will be half the fat content of the original, so their fat levels can still be quite high.

One of my favourite dairy products for cooking is **half-fat crème fraiche**. At around 14g per 100ml, that works out at just over 2g fat for every tablespoon. I whisk this crème fraiche into a quick pan sauce or trickle it over my pasta or into a baked potato.

If I want something even lower-fat, I use 8% **fromage frais** (almost half as much fat again) or the ultimate 0% fat fromage frais.

The same principle applies with **natural yogurts**.

There are varying levels of 'low fat', so check the label to be sure if you are following a strict weight loss programme.

However, be aware of the difference between a low-fat product (the lowest category) and one described as lower-fat or reduced-fat, which will simply have a lower fat level than the full-fat version. The wording on packaging can be misleading. A product described as 92% fat-free means that it will have 8% fat – not quite as lean as one is led to believe.

Sheep's and goat's milk products In recent years we have seen a tremendous variety of dairy products made with these milks and delicious they are too. Basically the same principles apply but sheep's milk is richer at just under 7% fat for whole milk, which gives it a slightly sweeter taste.

Cheese

Cheeses are literally concentrated milk products, and they all have high fat levels. However, for vegetarians they are not only good sources of protein but rather useful in cooking! But take it easy all the same or try lower-fat versions.

> *Be aware of the difference between a low-fat product and one described as lower-fat or reduced-fat.*

Hard cheeses For example, Cheddar cheese has a fat level of 34%, which varies very slightly according to maturity. Parmesan cheese on the other hand has 28% of fat per 100g and because it is sold full flavoured, well matured and easy to grate finely, it is brilliant for weight-reducing dishes as you need much less for a good cheesy flavour. I love it and buy a small block of the best quality I can find, then freshly grate a little at a time. For the best quality, look for the green and red striped stamp with the words 'Parmigiano Reggiano' on the pack or engraved in red dots on the rind.

Soft cheeses Here again fat levels vary enormously. Cream cheeses (including Philadelphia, French garlic soft cheese such as Boursin and Italian mascarpone) are the highest at around 40% fat, followed by curd cheese (also 'lite' cream cheese) at 16%, ricotta at 14%, cottage cheese at around 4%, whilst low-fat cottage cheese and quark (skimmed-milk soft cheese) are a saintly 0.2%. Incidentally, quark is an excellent, versatile soft cheese for cooking, particularly in lower-fat cheesecakes and salad dressings.

Cooking with lower-fat products

In general, lower- and low-fat dairy products do not cook well.

Half-fat cheese does not melt evenly and goes 'clumpy' when heated.

Low-fat yogurts and **fromage frais** tend to separate out and look curdled when heated. Try whisking them first with a little flour or stirring them into a dish after it has been cooked, or simply spoon a dollop or two on top just before serving. This looks particularly attractive if sprinkled with chopped fresh herbs or a good pinch of spice.

The exception to this is **crème fraiche** – even half-fat crème fraiche will whisk into a hot dish without curdling; it is something to do with the production process. But check labels of reduced-fat crème fraiche – some brands contain gelatine as thickeners.

Fat percentage levels in dairy products

Milk:
whole milk 4%
semi-skimmed or half-fat milk just under 2%
skimmed milk 0.1%

Cheese:
cream cheeses 40%
Cheddar 34%
fresh parmesan 28%
soft goat's cheese 16%
cottage cheese 4%
skimmed-milk soft cheeses 0.2%

Cream and yogurts:
double cream 48%
crème fraiche 40%
half-fat crème fraiche 23%
single cream 18%
fromage frais between 8% and almost 0% fat
Greek and whole-milk yogurts 10%
low-fat yogurts 0.1–2.3%
buttermilk 0.2%

FATS AND OILS

There is no doubt about it, fats and oils do make our food palatable. The good news is that we need a certain amount of fat in our diet to help some of our body functions. But nowhere near as much as we all eat at the moment. Some fatty acids help in the growth and repair of cell structures and are good sources of vitamins A, D, E and K. But fats and oils are huge sources of energy – they can supply over twice the amount of energy found in carbohydrate foods, for example.

The 'danger' of all fats – and sugars – is the fact that they

> *We need a certain amount of fat in our diet to help some of our body functions. But nowhere near as much as we all eat.*

are present in so many processed foods, which we can be blissfully unaware of. Biscuits, cakes and snack foods may be obvious sources, but watch out for pizzas, ready-made sauces, salad dressings, vegetarian 'mock meat' products (e.g. sausages and burgers), pies, pasties and crispy-crumbed products. Even if you eat them with a salad or vegetables in the mistaken belief you're having a nice lean meal, the opposite may be true. The best guideline is to check the packaging label.

How much should we eat?

For everyday weight maintenance, cut your fat intake by a third.

However, if you are trying to lose weight, you should halve it or, better still, cut out all but small amounts of the healthier fats and oils.

Here is a reminder:

Daily fat levels
Normal fat levels Adult men should aim for no more than 99g fat per day; adult women 77g fat per day.
To lose weight Reduce your fat levels to at least 85g a day for men and 67g for women.

WHAT ARE HEALTHIER FATS AND OILS?

Much has been written about good fats and so-called bad fats.

Saturated fats are thought to increase harmful blood cholesterol levels. In general they remain hard at room temperature. As a vegetarian, you will not be interested in meat fats. But saturated fats are still present in egg yolks, whole milk (silver top and

Jersey), cream, butter and cheese, and there are also a few vegetable saturated fats, like coconut, so beware.

We should keep our saturated fat levels to just 10% of our calorie intake. But **all** fats and oils are still high in calories.

'Healthier' fats are generally fats and oils that are liquid or very soft at room temperature. They have very low levels of saturates and are divided into two categories: **polyunsaturates** and **monounsaturates**.

Major sources are **vegetable oils**, such as olive, sunflower and soya oils, margarines and lower-fat spreads made with these oils. They are also found in peanuts and even avocados. These fats have a cleansing effect on the blood and help to maintain a healthy heart.

But gram for gram they still have the same calorific value as saturated fats, so if you aim to lose weight, **control your intake of all fats**.

Spreads, margarine and butter

Fat spreads can vary in fat content, from butter at 80% fat right down to very low-fat vegetable spreads at around 27% fat. The lower the fat content, the higher the water level, so low-fat spreads are fine for spreading on toast or crackers or whisking into sauces, but no good for baking. Spreads can be buttery-flavoured or have an olive oil base; what you choose is purely a matter of taste.

Butter has around 80% fat, half of which will be saturated fat. But the occasional teaspoonful whisked into a simple sauce or a dollop on top of a baked potato can be a heavenly treat.

Baking fats or shortenings will be almost 100% fat, which is why pastries should become occasional treats only! They will be made with vegetable oils, so are low in saturates but still very high in calories.

Fat content in fats and margarines:
butter 80%
baking margarine 80%
vegetable fat spreads 38–73%
very low-fat spreads 27%

SALAD OILS

Every tablespoon of oil of whatever type has around 120 calories.

Every tablespoon of oil of whatever type has around 120 calories. Sunflower is the best all-rounder, but you shouldn't be interested in using too much of any oil!

Groundnut oil, made from peanuts, is the oil favoured by Oriental cooks as it can be heated to high temperatures without burning, making it ideal for stir-frying.

Rapeseed, **soya** and **corn oils** are fine for cooking but I find the flavours a bit powerful for dressings. All these oils have high levels of polyunsaturates, which vary according to the vegetable source (check the label).

Olive oils are increasing on our supermarket and deli shelves at a rate that makes you wonder if they are all genuine. (Doesn't it take many years to grow olive trees?) I won't get into too much detail because your interest should be only on a need-to-know-basis! The greater percentage of European olive oil comes from Spain, where it is harvested and produced, but it could have been bottled in any other European country. If the country of origin concerns you (and the characteristics of the oil do vary according to country and region), check the label if you want to be sure.

Extra-virgin olive oil is classified by an acidity level of less than 1%. For a wonderful fruity aroma buy the best-quality extra-virgin olive oil you can afford; then you only need use a teaspoon or so at a time. You may even want to splash out on a single-grower olive oil, and if you are invited to taste extra-virgin olive oils, you will notice specific differences with flavours ranging from fruity through to peppery. Bottles sold simply as 'olive oil' or 'pure olive oil' are the next classification down and although they lack the flavour of extra-virgin oils they are excellent for cooking, albeit a trickle at a time.

AROMATIC OILS

You have noticed, I'm sure, an increasing array of slender bottles in deli and supermarkets featuring oils with various obscure names. Treat these as you would essential oils – that is, use them for their aroma and flavouring. Remember, they have the same calorie content as ordinary oils. They are not suitable for frying as they burn too easily and also they are expensive. But this of course is a plus for weight control because you only need a few drops to impart an exotic flavour. A little goes a long way.

Sesame seed oil is perhaps the best known. Again, buy a good ethnic brand name and make sure it has been made from roasted sesame seeds.

Nut oils – walnut, hazelnut and almond – are good trickled in half-teaspoonfuls over hot rice, potatoes or pasta, as well as being used in salad dressings.

Pumpkin seed oil is a newcomer with an intriguing flavour.

All these oils are pungent so use in small amounts. Store them all in the fridge as they can turn rancid if left at room temperature.

SUGARS

The subject of sugars can be confusing. We associate them with unhealthy 'bad' and fattening foods such as biscuits, cakes, confectionery and ice creams, yet in terms of actual calories sugars have the same value as apparently 'good' foods. The main problem with sugars is that we tend to eat them in combination with fats, or they are used in high amounts and so they appear to be high calorie. (The other big concern with sugars relates to dental care and the cravings that a sweet tooth gives us for sweet foods, but that's another issue.)

In small, modest and occasional amounts, sugar does you little harm. A teaspoon of sugar still only comes in at 15 calories, and a light dusting of icing or fine caster sugar even less. So, if you use sugars in these kind of amounts to make dishes more palatable, that is fine. A good pinch of sugar to a dressing, for example, or a dusting of icing sugar over tart, fresh fruit, or a teaspoonful of honey in a Chinese sauce are all in moderation and provide a good balance to recipes and flavours. Just remember that with pure sugar you get nothing else besides calories.

It helps to know a little about the types of sugars too. The white, sprinkly sugar we are all familiar with is **sucrose** – once labelled 'pure, white and deadly' and weighing in at just under 400 calories per 100g. But when sugar is used in high amounts, the calories begin to become more significant; for example, in jams, sugary drinks, baked goods, confectionery and so on. So those are the foods you must be aware of, not the occasional sprinkle or pinch of sugar.

The density of sugar matters too. Icing sugar is particularly useful if used lightly. Because it is so fine, it dissolves more quickly on our tongues and so tastes sweeter. A tablespoon of icing sugar weighs just 10g and yet can be scattered over a large bowl of strawberries to serve two or three people. Great calorie value!

> *In small, modest and occasional amounts, sugar does you little harm.*

Fructose, found in fruits, honey and tree syrups, is sweeter than sucrose but it seems to taste less sweet because it is diluted in water. However, when concentrated by drying, fruit sugars become quite intense in flavour, which is why currants and raisins taste so sweet and are actually quite high in calories. Honey is about a third lower in calories than sucrose at around 300 calories per 100g, but 1 tablespoon of honey weighs around 25g, which gives a figure of 75 calories, compared to 60 calories per tablespoon for ordinary sugar. I only mention it because there is this lingering idea that somehow honey is 'less fattening' than sugar. It isn't – it just tastes nicer. My favourite simple sweetener is maple syrup, a tablespoon of which contains around 40 calories.

Artificial sweeteners are substances hundreds of times

sweeter than sucrose, which is why they taste so sweet and why we use them in tiny, tiny amounts. They are sold as a neat compact pill, as a fine powder or in granulated powder form, and now can be bought mixed with sucrose as 'half-sugars'. They taste bitter if heated or used for cooking, so add afterwards. For example, stew fruits first, then add sweetener.

> **There is this lingering idea that somehow honey is 'less fattening' than sugar. It isn't – it just tastes nicer.**

Some people are affected by certain sweeteners, which cause them to develop headaches. If you are one of the few, then check the label.

CHAPTER FOUR

Full of Vim and Vit

VITAMINS AND MINERALS

A good working knowledge of vitamins and minerals is useful, whether you are planning on changing your diet to lose weight or setting up a new weight-maintenance style. This also explains why it is important to eat a good cross-section of foods even when you are dieting – rather than exclude any. Formula or magic-wand diets that are followed for too long may well be lacking in essential substances that we need to keep us healthy, with the result that we could end up lacking in energy and vulnerable to infections. Who wants to be thin and listless?

Judging from the mushrooming of the dietary supplement market, most of us are aware that our bodies need these vital compounds but I suspect that many of us prefer to pop pills as an easy option rather than take time to delve into why we would be better off with the 'real McCoy'. The best and purest forms are found in 'real' food, and nutritionists suggest supplements only for certain conditions such as pregnancy, old age and those with allergies or very fussy children.

Even if you cut down on your calorie intake overall, you must not decrease your intake of vitamins and minerals. In them-

> *It is important to eat a good cross-section of foods even when you are dieting – rather than exclude any.*

selves these nutrients are not 'fattening' so there is no reason why you cannot aim for a full complement, as near as possible. Even if certain vitamins occur widely in high-calorie foods, there is generally a lower-fat alternative.

Here is a basic summary.

VITAMINS

These are categorized as either fat-soluble or water-soluble.

Fat-soluble vitamins

Vitamin A This vitamin is also known as retinol. It is found in egg yolks, spinach, cresses, dried apricots and peppers. A substance called carotene, occurring in yellow and orange fruits and vegetables, is a precursor of vitamin A; in other words, our bodies can make a supply if we ingest carotene-rich foods, like carrots. It is good for bright eyes, breathing, a healthy digestion and infection-free bladders. It is also an antioxidant, one of the substances that can help protect against unstable free radicals, which may cause cancer.

> *A lack of vitamin D can make you irritable so if you start snapping at everyone, get out into the sunshine.*

Vitamin D This is often called the sunshine vitamin. Again our brilliant bodies can synthesize an internal supply as long as our skin is exposed to some sunlight each day. A good reason for taking healthy exercise. It is also found in fortified cereals and margarines. This vitamin helps the body absorb calcium and phosphorus. A lack of it can make you irritable so if you start snapping at everyone, get out into the sunshine.

Vitamin E This is another antioxidant, which maintains healthy cell membranes. The best sources are corn and sunflower oils, wheatgerm, tahini, peanuts, seeds and avocados. As these foods are also high in fats, you should watch your intake, but small amounts will still give you plenty of protection.

Vitamin K This vitamin, found in green leafy vegetables, seaweeds, vegetable oils and rich dark sugars, is good for the blood.

Water-soluble vitamins
Water-soluble means that these vitamins are rather vulnerable, as they can be washed or boiled away, or can decrease over time.

Vitamin B This is a large and complex group.
B1 (thiamin) is found in whole grains (including breads, pasta and rice), eggs, beans and peas. It helps release energy from carbohydrates. You need to take daily amounts of this vitamin as our bodies cannot store too much at one time. A lack of it makes us feel weak.
B2 (riboflavin) occurs in milk, cheese, eggs, green leafy vegetables, brewer's yeast, whole grains and wheatgerm. Another energy-associated vitamin, B2 is affected by light and heat, so don't leave your milk bottles on the doorstep for too long.
B6 (pyridoxine) helps our bodies utilize proteins, and prevents irritability and mouth ulcers. It is found in bananas, potatoes and pulses.
B12 is found in yeast extracts, soya milks, seaweeds, miso, breakfast cereals, eggs and dairy foods. Vegans will have to take B12 supplements or eat a lot of seaweed products.
Folic acid is important in the formation of cells and is now recommended for women planning pregnancy. But it is good for all of us in minimizing anaemia. Green vegetables, yeast extract, eggs and cereals are good sources.

Vitamin C This is the third antioxidant. It is vital for the formation of collagen in bones, muscles and skin, and assists in the absorption of iron from non-animal sources (important to vegetarians). A lack of vitamin C causes joint pains, poor teeth and slows the healing of wounds. Scientific studies still continue to investigate the claim that very high doses of vitamin C can prevent colds by boosting our immune systems. The best sources are citrus fruits, strawberries, kiwis, cherry juice, broccoli, parsley, frozen peas, blackcurrants and new potatoes. Vitamin C is also vulnerable to heat, so eat these foods raw or very lightly cooked. Make sure you have a good daily intake because our bodies can't store more than a day's supply at a time.

MIGHTY MINERALS

At first sight it seems a bit strange that we need inorganic substances associated with the earth and sea: iron, copper, calcium, selenium, zinc, fluoride, iodine, magnesium, phosphorus, sulphur and potassium. Which just goes to prove that we are all children of the soil. But, yes, they are also essential for the efficiency of our enzymes and hormones – in regulating blood clotting, heartbeat, digestion, bone formation and body fluids to name but a few.

Some minerals, which we need less of than others, are known as microminerals or trace elements but they are still vital for everyday well-being. They occur naturally in many of the same foodstuffs, so as long as you eat a good varied amount often, you won't go short.

Vegetarians should ensure that they eat good sources of iron-rich foods such as lentils, fortified breakfast cereals, seeds, soya products, pulses, eggs and dark green leafy vegetables such as spinach. But make sure that you also eat foods that are high in vitamin C, such as lemon juice, as your body needs vitamin C in order to utilize the iron.

Mineral-rich foods

These include: tofu, soya beans, soya mince, beans and pulses, green leafy vegetables (including spinach), broccoli, potatoes, swedes, parsley, whole grains, millet, oats, seaweeds, seeds (especially sesame and pumpkin), nuts (especially brazil nuts), prunes, apricots, dates, molasses or unrefined brown sugars, soya milks, bananas, wheatgerm and yeast extract.

CHAPTER FIVE

Flavour Without Fat

LEAN-LINE COOKING

I t does take a little time to adjust to cooking in a low-fat way but more and more of us are beginning to enjoy a leaner, less rich style of eating without pouring cream over puddings, cooking in a lot of butter or spreading it thickly on bread.

Simple things can help, like letting your slice of breakfast toast cool before spreading it. This helps cut the fat, because it won't sink in as it melts. Or adding a knob of butter or spread to vegetable water to give a buttery taste and sheen, then draining off the water as normal. You get a nice subtle flavour but use less fat than if you tossed cooked veggies with butter.

On page 129 you will find ideas for low-fat salad dressings.

One useful standby for cooking is the **virtually fat-free cooking spray**. It is useful for dry-frying and is sold in small aerosol cans. If you have a choice of sprays, buy the olive oil flavour. I find that garlic-flavoured sprays taste rather pungent but are quite good used on cubes of bread when making oven-crisp croutons (see page 128 for recipe).

To use, first heat a pan until hot, then spray the surface just before adding the food. You don't need to heat the spray itself – it just evaporates away. There are also hand-pumped olive oil sprays, which deliver a fine oily mist without suspicious additives.

Another good idea is the following recipe for a good, all-purpose, **lower-fat béchamel sauce**, using lower-fat spreads and skimmed milk. It has many uses – for example, poured over cooked chicken or fish – and it adds a light creaminess to pasta dishes and vegetables. The method is simplicity itself and there is no need to make a roux, as in a classic béchamel sauce, which could turn lumpy.

LOWER-FAT BÉCHAMEL SAUCE

Makes enough for 2–3 servings
Calories per portion/serving: 45

INGREDIENTS
300ml skimmed milk
1–2 level tablespoons flour (see method)
1 teaspoon olive oil vegetable spread
a light grating of fresh nutmeg
sea salt and freshly ground black pepper

METHOD
If you want a thin sauce, use 1 tablespoon of flour; for a thicker coating sauce, use 2 tablespoons.

Put the milk, flour and spread into a saucepan. Bring slowly to the boil, whisking or stirring continuously. Slowly it will come together as a smooth, thickened, creamy sauce. Simmer for 1 minute, season, then remove from the heat and allow to cool. Stir occasionally to stop a skin forming. That's it. Lastly add your chosen flavouring, from the box below.

Flavourings
- 2 teaspoons coarse-grained mustard and a dash or two of hot pepper sauce.
- 1 egg, hard-boiled and chopped, plus chopped fresh dill, parsley or chives.
- 1 tablespoon freshly grated parmesan cheese with $1/2$ teaspoon mustard powder.
- 1 small chopped onion, cooked in a little water for about 5 minutes until softened, plus a little grated parmesan cheese.
- A good fistful of chopped fresh parsley and chives for a classic green sauce.

POTS OF FLAVOUR

I have two shelves near my cooker that hold many different bottles and jars of sauces, relishes and vinegars. I reach for these when I want to add instant flavour with virtually no calories.

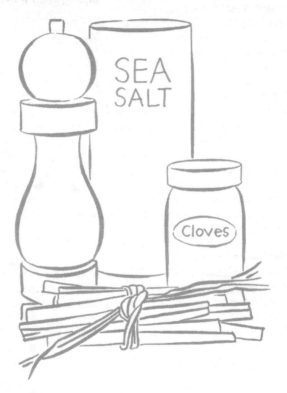

SAUCES

Soy sauces
With their balance of caramel-salty-aromatic flavours, these are indispensable for the vegetarian cook and ideal for a host of dishes, not just Oriental. A few shakes can make such a

difference to even the simplest vegetable mixture, stirred into a bowl of rice, or shaken over boiled potatoes. But do buy a good Chinese or Japanese brand for the best flavour (e.g. Lee Kum Kee, Sanchi or Kikkoman). These are naturally brewed soy sauces with a salty-sweet full flavour.

Soy sauces are indispensable for the vegetarian cook and ideal for a host of dishes, not just Oriental.

Tamari
This is a gluten-free soy sauce favoured by those interested in wholefood cooking. Use light soy sauce for dressings, and sprinkle over grilled vegetables, rice or noodles. It's also divine beaten into eggs for an omelette. Dark soy sauce is best in richer sauces, bean pots or soups.

Vegetarian 'oyster' sauce
This is made not with oysters but an extract of shiitake mushrooms.

Mushroom ketchup
This good old-fashioned sauce is similar to vegetarian 'oyster' sauce and is very useful for adding flavour. It is excellent added to bean stews or shaken into stir-fries, etc. Good too sprinkled over eggs and pasta.

Note: I have not included Worcestershire sauce in any recipes because it contains a small amount of anchovy. If, however, you are a fish-eating vegetarian, you will find it a useful flavouring.

MUSTARDS

Coarse-grained mustards are good in rich-flavoured bean and root vegetable casseroles. And, of course, mixed with a teaspoon of clear honey, they are great in dressings. Blend with a little fromage frais for a punchy baked potato filling.

Dijon mustard is a tangy, yellow-brown, smooth mustard full of flavour without fiery heat, good again as a background flavouring.

English mustard is bright yellow, sold as a loose powder or ready-made in pots. A light dusting of English mustard powder is good sprinkled onto dried breadcrumbs to use as a crunchy topping.

Mild American mustard (sold under the name of French's) is just right for lean veggie burgers.

STOCK CUBES AND POWDERS

Ideally it would be wonderful to use freshly made stock for every suitable occasion. Sometimes I do take the time to make a vegetable stock for spectacular soups and special sauces. But in general I use the Marigold brand of vegetable stock powder (they also make a vegan version) or vegetable stock cubes by Knorr or Just Bouillon. These brands don't seem to have the artificial whiff associated with some stock cubes or powders.

If I need to add dark colour, a dash or two of gravy browning suffices (it's made from caramel) and of course soy sauce is a good flavour enhancer.

But simple water often makes a light and simple liquor, especially when it comes to delicate cream vegetable soups. The best carrot soup I ever had was made simply with carrots, water, a little onion and lemon juice. These ingredients delivered a pure, wholesome flavour with few calories.

HOME-MADE VEGETABLE STOCK

There may be occasions when you would like to make a batch of fresh stock for a special soup, sauce or casserole. It is very easy to do and freezes well. Use button mushrooms for a light colour, larger open ones for a darker stock. If you have any leftover dry white wine, add a large glass to the pot whilst it simmers away for extra flavour.

INGREDIENTS

1 large onion, peeled
1 small head garlic, halved crossways
2 large carrots, chopped roughly
2 sticks celery, chopped
1 large leek, chopped roughly
1 red or yellow pepper, halved and seeded
about 150g mushrooms
about 3–4 overripe tomatoes, quartered
2 bay leaves
1 large sprig fresh thyme
handful fresh parsley stalks
1/2 teaspoon black peppercorns
1 teaspoon fresh coriander berries

METHOD

Simply put all the vegetables into a very large saucepan. Pour on enough cold water to reach about 4cm above the top of the vegetables. Add the herbs, peppercorns and coriander.

Bring slowly to the boil, then lower to a gentle simmer, uncovered, for about 20 minutes. Leave to get quite cold, even overnight, so that the vegetables steep in the liquor.

Strain. You should get about 2 litres of a golden-coloured stock. Use this fresh or freeze in 500ml blocks. **Note**: no salt is added at this stage. You can add salt when using the stock in a recipe.

RELISHES AND CHUTNEYS

These will be high in sugar, but generally low in fat or oils, so you can use with caution. Old-fashioned chutneys such as mango, plum or green tomato can be spread a teaspoon at a time in sandwiches in place of butter or spread. They are good too with cottage cheese.

But there are now many new-wave relishes in the food stores from the Americas and Asia – all well worth using in cooking, again a small spoonful at a time. Try a mild **chilli relish** stirred into a stew of red kidney beans or spooned into a baked potato instead of butter or cheese. With **Indian relishes** you may have to check on fat levels as sometimes they can be high in oil or ghee (clarified butter). **Thai relishes** and sauces tend to be quite runny and are great for trickling over a bowl of rice or using as a dipping sauce for vegetable crudités. Look for bottles of sweet chilli sauce or relish.

VINEGARS

Lots of flavour and zilch calories. Vinegars vary in acidity and flavour, so it is worth having two or three different types. The most useful I find is **rice wine vinegar**, which is light, fragrant and not at all overpowering, good for sprinkling neat over salads.

Alternatively, if you can find it, buy the ready-made sushi dressing called **seasoned rice wine vinegar**. Otherwise make up your own mix with 100ml rice wine vinegar heated gently with 1 tablespoon salt and 1 tablespoon caster sugar. Store in a small screw-topped jar. It's really nice over a big bowl of cold, crisp iceberg lettuce tossed with fresh herbs and a few pinches of toasted sesame seeds.

Cooks also use **basalmic vinegars** in hot dishes or mixed half and half with a lighter wine vinegar for

> *Relishes and chutneys will be high in sugar, but generally low in fat or oils, so you can use with caution.*

dressings. These vinegars are from the Modena area of Italy, and are matured in a variety of wood barrels over a period of years. The longer the maturation time, the better the quality and depth of flavour. So buy the best quality you can afford because a bottle lasts a long time. I have tasted basalmic vinegars costing over £100 (only a little sip, I hasten to add) but the flavour was sensational. Basalmic vinegar has a host of delicious uses in lean cuisine. Sprinkle over vegetables, ratatouille or pasta or make a red onion relish with slow-cooked red onion slices, a little brown sugar, crushed garlic and 1–2 tablespoons of

> *Balsamic vinegar has a host of delicious uses in lean cuisine.*

basalmic vinegar. It's also sensational dribbled over a dish of sliced strawberries.

Sherry vinegar has an oaky, sweet aroma and is becoming increasingly popular. It is sold in half-bottles. A trickle or two gives a mild spicy flavour to dressings.

Wine vinegars – red, white or champagne – are good all-purpose flavourings, which I often mix half and half with full-flavoured vinegars. These are the vinegars that chefs use sometimes when deglazing a pan after pan-frying, to cook off the moisture by reducing it down to concentrate the flavour.

Fruit vinegars, such as raspberry or blackcurrant, are invariably wine vinegars that have had soft fruits steeped in them for a period of weeks, then strained off. It's easy to make your own should you have a glut of berries. Or you could poke sprigs of fresh herbs or long thin chillies into bottles of white wine vinegar. Add a few whole spices like peppercorns or cloves or cinnamon for added flavour. It is advisable to heat the vinegar first to boiling point to pasteurize the herbs and intensify the flavour. Cool before rebottling.

Cider vinegar is wonderfully apple-y and a great favourite of mine in long, slow, winter-style stews, but it is quite strong and sharp. I like it mixed with coarse-grained mustard and a teaspoon of clear honey to toss into hot, fresh pasta, or sprinkled over dry-fried smoked tofu.

Vinegar strengths

The mildest are rice wine vinegars, followed by wine vinegars, sherry and basalmic vinegars, malt vinegars and lastly cider vinegars. Malt vinegars are used in pickles or found in sprinkler bottles in chip shops!

CHAPTER SIX

Lean, Green, Store Cupboard Foods

T here are an increasing number of dried, bottled or tinned ingredients that a healthy vegetarian wishing to lose weight can buy and store. These add flavour (with the minimum of calories) to vegetables, pulses, low-fat dairy foods and fruits.

DRIED MUSHROOMS

Mushrooms naturally have a very high water content, so when they are dried not only do they shrink right down but their flavour intensifies greatly, which makes them very useful in cooking. And, like fresh mushrooms, they are very low in calories. All you need to do to rehydrate is soak them in warm water (just enough to cover) for 15 minutes or so. Use the soaking water too for flavour.

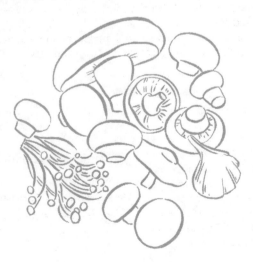

There are many varieties of dried mushrooms, mostly the woodland type, which are full-flavoured. Most popular are the French **ceps**, which Italians call porcini. Other European mushrooms include **morels** and **chanterelles**. Japanese and Chinese mushrooms are called **shiitakes**. These have quite an Oriental flavour, but are equally great in Western-style stews and casseroles. When soaked, you'll need to cut off the stalks, which make tough eating. All dried mushrooms look fearfully expensive, but a little goes a long way. Once soaked, treat as fresh.

SUN-DRIED TOMATOES

A good quality sun-dried tomato will have the most wonderfully sweet, full and fruity flavour. Sadly many on sale in supermarkets are either packed in oil (which makes them quite prohibitively calorific) or are rather dried and brittle. The best shops from which to buy sun-dried tomatoes are good-quality Italian delis. They can be so moist and concentrated that it is almost like eating a raisin.

Pliable dried tomatoes can be snipped into dishes or over salads, but in the main, they are best if soaked first in warm water for 20 minutes. As with mushrooms, the soaking water can be used like a stock.

I have on occasion seen sun-dried peppers and aubergines sold alongside tomatoes. Treat them in the same way.

SEAWEEDS/SEA VEGETABLES

The growth of sushi and noodle bars in the West has made us more aware of Japanese foods and, in particular, packs of various dark green dried seaweeds. Highly nutritious, they provide valuable sources of vitamins and minerals whilst adding flavour and colour to a host of different dishes from soups and salads to stir-fries and sushi.

Dried seaweeds provide valuable sources of vitamins and minerals whilst adding flavour and colour.

Seaweeds are cultivated around the coasts of Japan, not simply dredged up from any old bay or sea! Dried seaweeds need to be soaked for about 15 minutes in warm water prior to use.

The mildest is **arame** with a mild nutty flavour. **Kombu** is used in small pieces as a flavouring for broths or for cooking with rice. **Nori** sheets are used for sushi or are lightly toasted and crushed as a garnish. **Wakame**, the sweetest in flavour, is the most popular and versatile. It can even be crumbled dry over dishes, just like grated cheese or chopped fresh herbs.

There are European seaweeds too – **samphire** is an old British favourite, harvested around salt marshes, as is **laverbread** from Wales. The French use varieties of seaweed too, such as **dulse**.

Do give seaweeds a try – not only is their calorie value is very low but they are bursting with all sorts of nutritional goodies.

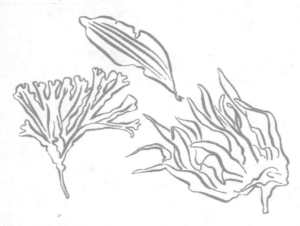

DRIED FRUITS

Drying intensifies the natural sweetness in fruits, which makes dried fruits useful on two counts. One: they are healthy sources of minerals and fibre, and two: they satisfy any cravings for sweet little nibbles. But dried fruits are still moderately high in calories so go easy on them. Remember, too, that they do not contain vitamin C. Raisins, currants and sultanas have around 250 calories per 100g; apricots and prunes contain around half that, at about 150 calories, because they have a higher moisture content.

Large dried fruits (**apricots, prunes, figs**) are good sources of fibre. In addition, **apricots** are high in beta carotene (for vitamin A) and iron. **Figs** are a good source of calcium, and **prunes** contain magnesium plus moderate amounts of other useful minerals.

So, a daily nibble of 4–6 apricots, figs or prunes or a small handful of currants or raisins should give you a nice sweet healthy treat.

Note: by dried fruits, I mean those that have been simply dried and concentrated in flavour, not those coated in sugar syrup or candied.

Fat-free baking fruit purées
You may have seen purées of prunes or apricots on sale as substitutes for fats in baking. This is a great idea, and they work well for cakes and chewy bars where you need a nice moist texture. They are not suitable, however, if you want a short texture as in crisp pastry, and as they are not very low in calories, use them judiciously.

HERBS AND SPICES

Eating in a lower-calorie way does not mean cooking with no flavour. As you learn to cook in a leaner, lighter way, you will begin to appreciate the great benefits of including herbs and spices, not just in special dishes but in a host of everyday ways. But for the best flavour, make sure you use them within the use-by dates.

> *As you learn to cook in a leaner, lighter way, you will begin to appreciate the great benefits of including herbs and spices.*

Whilst there are some general guidelines about which herbs and spices suit certain foods, do feel free to experiment. Start with a small collection (listed here as Useful Basics) and then build up if you feel the need.

HERBS

Fresh herbs are now a regular feature of supermarkets and you can find them in almost any month of the year. Small packs of a few sprigs or leaves may look expensive but they should do two or three meals and they will keep for a good week, if resealed in their packs at the bottom of the fridge.

Herbs such as **parsley**, **coriander**, **mint** and **dill** (which are nicest and healthier when used in fistfuls rather than in cautious pinches) are best bought in bunches. Halal butchers are a good source of supply if you have one in your area. If their bunches of herbs look a bit bedraggled, steep them in a bowl of cold water, drain well and store in the fridge wrapped loosely in a large food bag. They soon regain their succulent sprigginess. Fresh growing herbs, however, should not be stored in the fridge. Keep those on a semi-shaded windowsill and water them occasionally.

Dried herbs have a shelf life too because the natural aromas do fade in time. Store them out of sunlight in a dry cupboard and once they start to go grey – replace! Otherwise you end up with a substance that looks and tastes like old grass clippings.

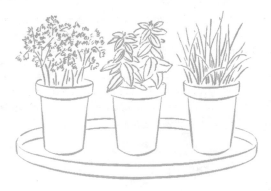

Useful Basic Herbs

Bay and kaffir lime leaves Although from different parts of the world (Europe and Thailand), these leaves can be used in similar ways. They add great flavour to any stew, casserole or milk pudding, and can be skewered on kebab sticks alternating with vegetables. The dried leaves have more flavour than fresh.

Chives They provide a mild oniony flavour (without the tears that come from chopping onions). Easy to snip over pasta dishes, salads or hot potatoes, and great stirred into low-fat soured creams, soft cheeses, etc. Not worth buying dried. Use salad onion tops if you can't find fresh chives.

Leaf coriander Both the fresh leaves and the stalks are used in Asian and Oriental cooking. Its leaves will wilt if not kept damp and bagged. Whole sprigs are good used in salads or in Mexican cooking.

Dill The fresh, feathery leaves are nice with hard-boiled eggs or rice, or when snipped over new potatoes. Good too with cauliflower and cabbage. Dill weed, the dried version, is fairly piquant. Dill seeds are really quite pungent, and best used in pickles.

Lemon grass This is a pale, lemon-scented, bulbous stalk with a flowery fragrance. Chop finely to add to Thai dishes or salad dressings. Good too cooked with milk puddings.

Mint A very useful, all-purpose herb, which gives a fresh Middle Eastern flavour to leafy salads if chopped roughly with parsley and a little dill. Essential and refreshing in Tabbouleh, and nice too with hot green beans.

TABBOULEH

Serves 2
Calories per portion/serving: 125

INGREDIENTS
75g bulghur wheat
2 tablespoons fresh lemon juice
1 tablespoon olive oil
half a mug chopped parsley
2 tablespoons chopped mint
1 tablespoon chopped fresh dill (optional)
2 salad onions, chopped
2 ripe tomatoes, chopped
sea salt and freshly ground black pepper

METHOD
Put the wheat into a large bowl and cover with cold water. Leave to soak for about 20 minutes, then drain well in a colander, pressing down with the back of a ladle or wooden spoon.

Return to the bowl and mix in the lemon juice, the oil, the herbs, the salad onions and the tomatoes. Season well with sea salt and lots of freshly ground black pepper. Cover and chill for 30 minutes, then serve.

Oregano and marjoram These classic Mediterranean herbs have many uses. They are easiest bought dried and are perhaps the only leafy herbs worth buying in this form, as the flavours are more concentrated. A must in pasta sauces or sprinkled over pizza. Good too with all vegetables. Marjoram is a more demure cousin, nice in omelettes.

Parsley The flat-leaf kind is for general use and garnishing, the curly leaf for flavour. A good source of vitamin C. Don't waste the stalks as they can be used too. Whole leaves are great in salads. Don't buy this herb dried – it has no flavour.

For a great flavour, snip tender sprigs of rosemary over roasted vegetables.

Rosemary and thyme These are both woody and pungent herbs, so they have similar uses. Like sage, sprigs of both can be dried. For a great flavour, snip tender sprigs of rosemary over roasted vegetables or ratatouille. Pinch tips of thyme and scatter over eggs, tomatoes and mushrooms.

Sage This is very pungent, so use sparingly. Good with broad beans, eggs and in Mediterranean recipes. It can be dried at home and then crushed into food, so if you don't use a whole pack or pot in a week, dry your own – don't waste it.

Tarragon This is one of the aniseed herbs. Strip the long thin leaves from a sprig; as it is a pungent herb, a little is all you need. A classic with eggs, cheese and cauliflower. Good too steeped in vinegar, which is nice trickled over salads instead of high-oil dressings.

SPICES

As with dried herbs, remember that spices have a shelf life, and should be stored out of direct sunlight. They can all lose their aroma with time.

The most commonly used spices are salt and pepper.

Salts These are the most used flavouring although we should all try to cut down on them. **Sea salt** has the purest flavour (so you need less); **table salt** has a distinctive aftertaste that is unpleasant. **Rock salt** goes into the cookpot (for vegetables, pasta and rice) and salt mills. **Fine crystal salt** is for sprinkling, whilst **coarse salt crystals** are wonderful for crushing over food. I appreciate that it may sound extravagant but in the great design of things, even sea salt is relatively inexpensive for the return on flavour.

Peppercorns It is possible to buy a colourful selection of these. They start green and ripen through to black. White peppercorns are black corns stripped of their casing – very fiery and pungent.

Three-Michelin-starred chef, Gordon Ramsay, taught me to mix whole spices with peppercorns for grinding in a pepper mill and I now have three different mixes to add a variety of flavourings – see below. (You need to break up larger whole spices, such as star anise or cinnamon before adding to the pepper mill.) The Chinese aromatic red Sichuan peppercorns are a particular favourite, especially ground over poached eggs.

AROMATIC PEPPER MIXES

Spice up your food by blending a personal mix of peppercorns for your pepper mill. Maximum flavour with zero calories!

BASE SPICE INGREDIENTS
3 tablespoons black peppercorns
3 tablespoons white peppercorns
1 tablespoon whole coriander berries

ADDITIONAL SPICES
1 teaspoon whole cloves
1 tablespoon Sichuan red peppercorns
1 teaspoon green cardamom pods
3 star anise, broken in pieces
1 large cinnamon stick, broken
1 teaspoon yellow and black mustard seeds

METHOD
Simply mix the base spices together in a bowl, adding one or more from the list of additional spices. Store what you don't use for the pepper mill in a small screw-topped jar.

Useful Basic Spices

Cinnamon Cinnamon sticks add flavour to casseroles, but you can break them into smaller pieces and add them to rice during cooking along with a couple of whole cloves and cardamoms.

Ground cinnamon is great used in Eastern Mediterranean dishes with lemons, turmeric, coriander and cumin. It is also good lightly sprinkled over fruit salads or more generously over rice puddings.

Ground coriander Dried ground coriander, made from the dried seeds, is mild, with a slightly citrus, musky flavour, which adds a slightly exotic, aromatic (but not hot) flavour to food. A very versatile spice – good with eggs, dressings, rice and roasted vegetables, and it combines well with cumin.

As an alternative to the powder, you can buy whole seeds and crush them lightly in a pestle and mortar.

Cumin This is sold either as whole seeds or ground, and both are indispensable to the adventurous cook. It is one of the milder, aromatic curry spices used in Indian and Chinese dishes, but good too in Mexican cooking combined with ground coriander and oregano. The seeds are nice when lightly dry-roasted and sprinkled over vegetables or new potatoes.

Garlic Garlic is well known but generally not used enough, to my mind. If you find garlic too pungent, boil a few cloves in a little water or roast a whole head, then pop the pulp out of the skins into a small dish and mash with a fork. Spoon into a small screw-topped jar and cover with a little sherry to store. Use within 1 week. When in season, the heads of large plump fresh garlic are quite heavenly.

To make garlic purée: simply peel the outer skin of the whole head and chop the rest up. Blend to a purée with some salt, store it in the fridge and use it all within 1 week. Alternatively, freeze in small amounts, say 1 tablespoon at a time.

Ginger The fresh roots keep a long time, bagged and stored at the bottom of the fridge. Buy large fleshy roots because although you only use a small amount each time, root ginger does keep well. If the flesh has gone woody, discard it. Break off a 2–3cm knob for each dish and peel thinly. Then either grate or cut into thin slivers and chop. It is good not only in Asian and Oriental food but also in stews, casseroles and soups made with carrots or parsnips.

Dried ground ginger is very pungent and is really only suitable for cakes and other baking, which of course you should not be interested in!

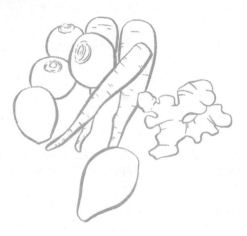

Nutmeg Keep a pot of whole nutmegs and a small, very fine grater, and grate it freshly. Nutmeg is a cook's best buddy, as it enhances so many foods. It is best over creamy sauces and milk puddings, but a light dusting is also good over crisp hot cabbage, potatoes, spinach, pasta and light cheesy dishes.

Nutmeg is a cook's best buddy, as it enhances so many foods.

Turmeric This bright, bright yellow spice is mildly aromatic and has a very mild flavour. It is a staple of curry mixes. Use a tiny amount, just 1/4 teaspoon at a time, otherwise it can become a little bitter. Nice with cheese, cauliflower and root vegetables, especially potatoes. It stains strongly, so take care.

Vanilla pods Long, thin and black, these are mostly used in puddings. Slit a pod in half lengthways and scrape out the minuscule seeds inside. Mix into milk that is heating for puddings or real custard and add the scraped-out pod also. The liquid will turn speckled. The whole pod can be removed before serving.

Very pungent spices These include **whole cloves**, **green cardamoms** and **star anise**. Use sparingly. They all keep for years, stored out of sunlight.

SPROUTING BEANS AND SEEDS

One of my first cookery books, for a major supermarket, was on rice, beans and pasta. Like all keen, eager novices I got terribly enthusiastic about my subject. One of the spin-offs was discovering the joys of sprouting my own beansprouts, which I have been doing ever since. Although many health food shops sell fresh sprouted pulses, there's little to beat sprouting your own. It is very easy and highly healthy. If you have children, you might like to give them the daily task of rinsing before they go to school. It's all part of the learning process.

Fresh beansprouts are very healthy and very low in calories. I find all sorts of uses for them, from tossing into salads, adding to stir-fries, stews and sauces, to even sprinkling on top of risottos and pastas instead of grated cheese or nuts. Not only are they a good source of protein and fibre, but as new plant life they are full of vital vitamins.

You need to allow 3–4 days for each batch to grow, but as this

> *Fresh beansprouts are very healthy and very low in calories.*

becomes part of your routine you'll find there is always a 'crop' on the go. I bought myself a special sprouting tray, which was very cheap and is now a good few years old. But to start with you can use old jam jars.

Most beans and seeds are suitable but they should be well within their sell-by date. Buy packs from a shop with a high turnover and check the pack dates etc. Allow 2–5 days for germinating and growing – sprouts are ready when they are at least three times the length of the original bean or seed.

Sprouting times

- Alfalfa and fenugreek seeds 2 days
- Lentils (Puy and larger Continental but not split red lentils) 2–3 days
- Mung and soya beans 3 days
- Chickpeas and aduki beans 3–4 days
- Flageolet and haricot beans 3–5 days

This is what you do

- Put 2–3 tablespoons of your chosen beans or seeds into a bowl and cover with lots of tepid water. Leave to soak overnight, then drain. Place in a large jam jar or the tray of a sprouting rack.
- If using a jam jar, cover the top with a circle of thin porous cloth, like a J-cloth or butter muslin, which you secure with an elastic band. Lay the jar on its side, shaking the beans to a single layer. Place the jar in a warm, semi-shaded spot so it is not in direct light. Leave for 12 hours.
- Run tepid water into the jar through the cloth top (without removing it), shake it gently and tip the water out – this rinses away the growing gases of the germinating beans. Lay the jar back again in position.
- Repeat this process twice a day until the beans or seeds start to sprout. When the sprouts are long enough, tip them out

into a colander, rinse again and store in a food container in the fridge, tucking into them as and when. They will keep like this, chilled, for about 3 days, by which time you will have started new batches.

- Do mix and match a variety of pulses and seeds. It is really cheap and fun to do, not to mention the great flavour and goodness they give you.

Note: if your beans or seeds haven't shown any signs of life after 2 days of rinsing, they are too old and should be discarded.

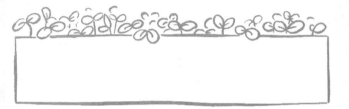

CHAPTER SEVEN

Enjoy What You Eat – For Ever!

BREAKFASTS

If there's one aspect of healthy eating that all nutritionists and diet gurus agree on, it's the importance of eating breakfast. Yet, for many of us watching our weight, it seems to be the one meal that we try to cut out in the mistaken belief that somehow we should save up our calorie allowance for later in the day. Well, nothing could be further from the truth and there are two good reasons for having at least something to eat after the long night fast.

1) Foods consumed at the start of the day when we are alert and full of go are utilized more efficiently by our bodies than the same amount of calories taken at night when we are relaxed and sleepy.
2) When we awake, our blood sugar levels are low after almost twelve hours without food. If our minds and bodies are to function to the best of their ability, we should be stoking up those energy levels. Otherwise, come mid-morning, we start to flag and snack on the wrong high-calorie, high-fat foods.

Breakfast foods are fortunately the right type for optimum health – cereals or toast, high in starchy complex carbohydrates, with fruits, modest proteins and lower-fat dairy products. We only need a small bowl of low-sugar, high-fibre cereal moistened with a small glass (125ml) of half-fat or skimmed milk for a nicely balanced 200 calories. Even a couple of pieces of brown toast spread thinly with a lower-fat spread, Marmite or honey will suffice, washed down with a glass of pure fruit juice.

If you really can't face eating first thing in the morning, wait a good hour or so and try again. Alternatively, pack a breakfast to eat en route to work. Try a brown bread sandwich of banana and honey or (thinly spread) peanut butter accompanied by a small carton of orange juice. A tub of low-fat 'live' yogurt with an apple or banana is as easy to eat at an office desk as a huge-calorie fistful of biscuits, a pack of crisps or a chocolate bar.

For a more leisurely breakfast, one or two poached eggs, or a large flat mushroom brushed with a whisper of olive oil and grilled nestled on brown toast with a shake or two of soy sauce, are truly delicious, not to mention my favourite, Squashy Tomatoes on Pesto Toast (page 94).

Perhaps the best breakfast, which is remarkably easy to get together, is a bowl of microwave porridge – it takes less time to heat up than having a shower. Make it with water and skimmed milk and serve with a trickle of maple syrup, runny honey or a light sprinkle of Billington's unrefined muscovado sugar – heaven in a bowl. Good too with a handful of juicy raisins or a sliced banana. I have two very lean healthy friends who eat this porridge every morning, winter and summer. They make a big batch every other day and reheat it in the microwave.

MICROWAVE PORRIDGE

Serves 1
Calories per portion/serving: 160
Cook and eat in the same bowl – choose a deep-sided one, with at least 500ml capacity (small pudding basin size).

Half-fill a teacup with instant porridge oats (ideally a variety with added bran). Tip into your chosen bowl and mix with a teacupful of skimmed milk and half a cupful of water. Stir well, cover with a saucer and cook on full power, timing according to the category of your microwave oven

- Category B/ 650 watts – 5 minutes
- Category D/ 750 watts – 4 minutes

If you have time, stir once halfway through; but if the bowl is deep-sided enough and your microwave has a turntable, you can skip this. Let the bowl stand for a couple of minutes before you stir again and tuck in.

If you have a less hearty appetite, you might like to try Breakfast in a Glass.

BREAKFAST IN A GLASS

Serves 1
Calories per portion/serving: 200
Scoop 1 (chilled) 140g tub of low-fat 'bio' yogurt into a blender with 1 small glass (125ml) of skimmed milk, 1 ripe banana (sliced) and any other soft fruit you may have lingering in the fridge or fruit bowl, such as a fistful of strawberries or a small, slightly wrinkled soft peach. Add 1 good tablespoon of dry porridge oats or 1 teaspoon each of wheatgerm and pure bran. Whizz to a cream and pour into a tall tumbler.

Once you have reached your ideal weight, there is no reason why you shouldn't treat yourself to a croissant or scrambled eggs on toast. Don't feel guilty about it, a little of

A little of what you fancy does you no harm, as long as it is little and not too often. Eating should be enjoyed!

what you fancy does you no harm, as long as it is little and not too often. Eating should be enjoyed!

QUICK LITE SCRAMBLED EGGS

Serves 1
Calories per portion/serving: 210

Scrambled eggs is a very personal dish. Only you know how you like them – runny or in soft billowing folds. Use only free-range or organic eggs for best flavour. I like to flavour mine with some aromatic pepper mix (page 82) or even some Chinese Sichuan red peppercorns plus a light dash of soy sauce. But it's the technique that makes this classic dish light and special.

- First, get your toast at the ready. Pop 2 slices of whole-meal or mixed grain bread into the toaster just as you are about to start cooking. If the bread is really fresh and flavoursome, there's no need to use even a low-fat spread.
- For each serving, beat 2 eggs with some sea salt (or soy sauce) and pepper. No milk. Put a small non-stick saucepan on to heat slowly and steadily and when you can feel a good heat rising, add just 1 teaspoon of olive or sunflower oil. Heat this for 30 seconds, then swirl it around the pan base and sides, and tip out any excess. Set the heat to medium-low.
- Pour in the beaten egg; it should sizzle as it hits the pan. Count to 10, then start to stir the edges, pulling lightly set egg from the sides into the middle. Wait another few seconds and again pull the sides into the middle as the egg sets. Continue like this until you have a creamy and lightly set egg – a total of some 2 minutes.
- By this time the toast will have browned so lay it on a plate. When the egg is just as you like it, and not a moment later or it will continue cooking and harden, spoon it on top of the toast and serve instantly – perfect scrambled eggs wait for no one.

LIGHT BITES

These quick and easy dishes are ideal as starters or light meals. If you want to lose weight rather than maintain your weight, follow the recipes with the halo (⌣) symbol.

MENU

Miso Plus
Squashy Tomatoes on Pesto Toast
Egg Foo Yong with Alfalfa Sprouts
Chickpea and Greek Salad Pitta
Spicy Yogurt and Mango Dip
Mashed Red Bean and Soft Garlic Cheese Sandwich
A Bowl of Bortsch
Gutsy Gazpacho
Velvety Broccoli Soup
Soufflé Omelette
Open-topped Hummus Snack Toasts
Spicy Aubergine Salsa with Pitta Melbas

MISO PLUS

Serves 1
Calories per portion/serving: 59 ⌣
Sachets of Japanese instant miso soup make excellent bases for light and healthy soups. Add whatever grated or chopped fresh vegetables you like. These are my favourites. Good with rice crackers.

INGREDIENTS

2 large button mushrooms
1 small carrot, scrubbed
small handful watercress sprigs or fresh coriander
1 sachet miso soup mix (e.g. Sanchi brand)
few shakes light soy sauce

METHOD
Thinly slice the mushrooms and coarsely grate the carrot. Place in a soup bowl. De-stalk the cress or coriander. Sprinkle over the soup mix and stir in a mugful of boiling water. Stir well and mix in the cress or herb leaves until they wilt. Shake over a little soy sauce to taste and drink.

SQUASHY TOMATOES ON PESTO TOAST

Serves 1
Calories per portion/serving: 190
A simple, classic snack. Choose a bread with seeds in it such as linseed. Don't use butter; instead, spread thinly with a good-quality pesto. Ripe plum tomatoes complete the plate.

INGREDIENTS
2 ripe tomatoes, preferably plum
sea salt and freshly ground black pepper
1 slice seeded, granary or wholemeal bread
2 teaspoons pesto sauce

TO SERVE
1 teaspoon sunflower seeds

METHOD
Preheat the grill. Halve the tomatoes lengthways and cut out the cores. Season and grill, cut side up, for 3–5 minutes until softened.

Toast the bread on both sides, then spread one side with pesto. Top with the tomatoes, squashing slightly with a fork. Scatter with the seeds, season again to taste and eat.

EGG FOO YONG WITH ALFALFA SPROUTS

Serves 1

Calories per portion/serving: 300

An ideal snack for using up leftover rice, preferably brown basmati. Ideally use spindly alfalfa sprouts, but ordinary mung beansprouts will do too.

INGREDIENTS

low-fat cooking spray
1 large egg
2 teaspoons light soy sauce
freshly ground black pepper
$^1/_2$ teaspoon sunflower oil
$^1/_2$ teaspoon sesame oil
1 small salad onion, chopped
about 4 heaped tablespoons cooked brown rice
2–3 tablespoons fresh alfalfa sprouts or mung beansprouts

TO SERVE

good pinch sesame seeds

METHOD

Heat a small non-stick frying pan until you feel a good heat rising, then spray lightly with low-fat cooking spray. Beat the egg with the soy sauce and pepper.

Pour in the egg and cook until lightly scrambled, but don't overcook. Remove the egg and break into chunks with a fork.

Reheat the pan again with the two oils and stir in the onion and rice. Cook until piping hot. Return the chunks of egg to the pan and mix in well, then stir in the sprouts and seasoning.

Sprinkle with sesame seeds and serve immediately.

CHICKPEA AND GREEK SALAD PITTA

Serves 1
Calories per portion/serving: 213
If you mix a grain food (e.g. pitta bread) with pulses (chickpeas), you have the ultimate well-balanced healthy meal.

INGREDIENTS
1 mini-size wholemeal pitta bread
1 medium ripe tomato
3cm length cucumber
1 salad onion
2 tablespoons low-fat natural yogurt
good pinch dried mint or dill
sea salt and ground black pepper
2 tablespoons canned chickpeas (or kidney beans), drained and
   rinsed

TO SERVE
squeeze fresh lemon juice

METHOD
Split the pitta bread open at the top. If you like it warm, pop into a toaster on a low setting for 1 minute or so to just heat through.

Meanwhile, chop the tomato, cucumber and onion quite finely and mix with the yogurt, mint or dill and seasoning.

Pile into the split pitta, spoon on the chickpeas, squeeze a little lemon juice on top and eat.

SPICY YOGURT AND MANGO DIP

Makes about 200ml (a small mugful)
Calories: 225
Make up a batch of this useful recipe to keep in the fridge so that you can dip into it whenever you feel a little peckish. Nice with sticks of carrot, cucumber or peppers. Alternatively, spoon

onto rice cakes and top with shredded radish, cucumber or grated carrot, and chopped mint.

INGREDIENTS
1 small onion, chopped finely
1 fat clove garlic, crushed
1 teaspoon olive or sunflower oil
good pinch cumin or black mustard seeds (optional but nice)
1 teaspoon curry powder
2 teaspoons mango chutney
150g tub very low-fat natural yogurt
sea salt and freshly ground black pepper

METHOD
Cook the onion and garlic in the oil with 1 tablespoon of water for about 5 minutes over a gentle heat until softened, stirring occasionally.

Add the cumin or mustard seeds and cook for a few seconds until you smell their aroma, then mix in the curry and mango chutney and cook for a few seconds more.

Remove from the heat and cool. When cold, stir in the yogurt and seasoning, then spoon into a pot and chill until required.

MASHED RED BEAN AND SOFT GARLIC CHEESE SANDWICH
....

Serves 1
Calories per portion/serving: 320
There are a number of low-fat soft cheeses now on sale with garlic and herb flavourings. They make excellent sandwich fillings, but don't go too wild as they are merely lower in fat, not fat-free. Here they are mixed with canned and mashed kidney beans and sandwiched between slices of your favourite wholesome and tasty fresh bread. No butter required.

INGREDIENTS
2 slices wholemeal, granary or seeded bread

1 tablespoon low-fat soft cheese with garlic and herbs, at room
  temperature
3 tablespoons red kidney beans, drained and rinsed
good pinch mild chilli powder, ground cumin or ground coriander
sea salt and freshly ground black pepper
1–2 teaspoons sunflower seeds (optional)
1 tomato, sliced thinly
few sprigs fresh watercress or parsley or coriander

METHOD

Spread the bread slices with the soft cheese. Mash the red beans
with a fork to a chunky purée and mix with the spices and seasoning.

Divide between the two slices and top with the seeds (if
using), tomato slices and sprigs of cress or fresh herbs. Season
again, then sandwich together and cut in quarters.

A BOWL OF BORTSCH
....

Serves 6
Calories per portion/serving: 60
Fresh beetroot makes fantastic soup that fills you up without
piling on the calories. You can leave it chunky or blend to a silky
purée. Eat with rye crispbreads for quick weight loss or (unbut-
tered) chunks of fresh wholemeal-style bread for weight maintenance. Make a big batch and freeze in single-portion sizes to
reheat in the microwave. See the box opposite for optional (but
nice) serving suggestions.

INGREDIENTS

500g raw beetroot
1 onion, chopped
2 fat cloves garlic, crushed
1 stick celery, chopped
1 tablespoon sunflower oil
1 teaspoon cumin seeds or 2
   teaspoons ground cumin
2 teaspoons ground coriander

> *Fresh beetroot
> makes fantastic
> soup that fills you
> up without piling
> on the calories.*

$^1/_2$ teaspoon dried thyme
1.5 litres water or vegetable stock (made with vegetable stock
    powder)
1 teaspoon sea salt
freshly ground black pepper

METHOD

Peel the beetroot thinly, then chop into small pea-size chunks.
(Use rubber gloves if you don't want pink-stained fingers.) Place
in a large saucepan with the onion, garlic, celery, oil and 3 tablespoons water. Heat until the pan starts to sizzle, then cover and
cook gently for 5 minutes or so, shaking the pan occasionally.

Stir in the spices and thyme and cook for another minute
then pour in the water or stock. Add the salt and pepper to
taste. Bring to the boil, then partially cover the pan and simmer
gently for 20 minutes, stirring once or twice.

If you like a smooth soup, blend in a food processor or
liquidizer; otherwise leave chunky. Serve with a choice of one of
the following serving suggestions, or all three.

Serving suggestions (per head)

- 2 button mushrooms, sliced thinly
- 1 tablespoon very low-fat natural yogurt
- sprinkling of chopped fresh parsley or chives

GUTSY GAZPACHO

· ·

Serves 2

Calories per portion/serving: 56 ☞

Made in a jiffy – no cooking required, so great for a hot summer.
Serve lightly chilled or pop a few ice cubes in the bowl. Add
finely chopped pepper and extra cucumber to add crispy bulk.

INGREDIENTS

3 large ripe plum tomatoes
1 red, green or yellow pepper

2 fat cloves garlic, peeled
2 teaspoons red wine vinegar
1/2 teaspoon sea salt
freshly ground black pepper
300ml water (or 150ml tomato juice plus 150ml water)

TO SERVE
6cm length cucumber, coarsely grated
a little chopped fresh parsley

METHOD
Quarter the tomatoes, cut out the cores, then chop the flesh. Core and seed the pepper; chop a third finely and set aside. Roughly chop the rest and place in a food processor with the garlic.

Whizz to a purée, then add the tomatoes, vinegar, salt and pepper to taste. Blend until smooth. With the blades still running, gradually pour in the water or juice and water.

Pour into a jug and chill until lightly cold. Check the seasoning again; cold food needs stronger flavours.

Pour into two chilled soup bowls and spoon in the reserved pepper, grated cucumber and parsley. Eat quickly. For a more substantial portion, have a chunk of warm crusty country-style bread, but no butter.

VELVETY BROCCOLI SOUP

Serves 4
Calories per portion/serving: 70
You will need a food processor for this. The idea is that you whizz the lightly cooked broccoli spears for what seems like ages until the mixture becomes a vibrant green and very, very smooth and silky. The texture is wonderfully creamy with hardly any fat.

INGREDIENTS
500g broccoli heads
1 onion, chopped
500ml skimmed milk

700ml light vegetable stock (can be
    made with stock powder)
sea salt and freshly ground black
    pepper

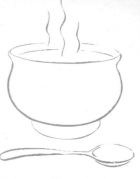

TO SERVE
2 tablespoons fat-free fromage frais

METHOD
Trim off the broccoli stalks and
chop finely. Chop up the florets,
keeping stalks and florets separate. Put the stalks and onion
into a saucepan with the milk, stock and seasoning.

Bring to the boil, then cover and simmer for 10 minutes until
just tender. Add the florets and continue cooking for another 5
minutes.

Strain the pan contents, keeping the liquid and solids separate. Put the vegetables into a food processor and blend for
what seems like ages, scraping down the sides a few times, until
you have a very smooth, almost glossy purée. You may have to
return some of the liquid to the food processor for the mixture
to blend smoothly.

Now with the blades whirring, slowly pour in the liquid and
continue to blend until the mixture becomes smooth. Pour
back into the pan and reheat gently to serve, checking the
seasoning. Serve with small dollops of fromage frais on top of
each bowl.

SOUFFLÉ OMELETTE
· ·

Serves 1
Calories per portion/serving: 200 (*including filling*)
A one-egg omelette is a sad sight, but a two-white, single-yolk
one whisked to a froth bulks out to a light yet filling meal. Egg
whites are lean and light; the yolks contain fat but they are very
nutritious. Serve plain with perhaps a few chopped herbs or add
a low-fat filling (choose one from the box below). Avoid cheese,

unless it's a single teaspoon of freshly grated parmesan. Nice with a mixed salad.

INGREDIENTS
2 large free-range eggs
good pinch dried thyme
sea salt and freshly ground black pepper
low-fat cooking spray

METHOD
First, choose and prepare your filling. Preheat a small to medium non-stick omelette pan until you can feel a good heat rising.

Meanwhile, separate one of the eggs and discard the yolk. Whisk the single egg white until it forms firm glossy peaks. In another bowl beat the whole egg with the thyme and seasoning to taste. Then, using a metal spoon, fold the beaten white into the whole egg.

Spray the hot pan with the cooking spray, then pour in the egg mixture. Cook gently until the base sets and the top dries out slightly, about 5 minutes.

Spoon the filling down one side of the omelette and, holding the pan over the serving plate, fold the other half over the filling. Then slide it all onto a plate and eat.

Filling suggestions
- 1 ripe tomato, chopped
- 3 button mushrooms, sliced thinly and poached in a little seasoned water, then drained
- 2 tablespoons sprouted lentils (see page 85), seasoned with soy sauce

---

OPEN-TOPPED HUMMUS SNACK TOASTS

Serves 1
Calories per portion/serving: 240
Use half-fat hummus as a snack base instead of butter, cream cheese, or even boring but worthy cottage cheese. Instead of ordinary salad cress, try the spicier mustard cress.

INGREDIENTS
2 rye crispbreads, rice cakes or Scandinavian snack rolls
2 level tablespoons reduced-fat hummus
1/4 punnet salad cress, snipped
1 small carrot, coarsely grated
2 teaspoons sunflower seeds or few pinches toasted sesame seeds
1–2 pinches mild chilli powder or sweet paprika
sea salt and freshly ground black pepper

METHOD
Spread the crispbreads, rice cakes or rolls with hummus and top with the cress, carrot, seeds, chilli or paprika and seasoning. Eat quickly so that the base remains crisp.

SPICY AUBERGINE SALSA WITH PITTA MELBAS

Makes about 300ml (a mugful), enough to serve 2
Calories per portion/serving: 210
A yummy dip with a low-fat creamy texture, popular in the Middle East.

INGREDIENTS
1 large firm aubergine
1 teaspoon olive oil
1 large sprig fresh rosemary
2 fat cloves garlic, sliced
sea salt and freshly ground pepper

1 tablespoon fresh lemon juice
good pinch cayenne or chilli powder
1 tablespoon natural low-fat yogurt (optional)
2 pitta breads

METHOD
Preheat the oven to 200°C, Gas Mark 6. Cut the aubergine in half, brush each side with the oil, place the rosemary and garlic on the cut sides and sandwich together. Cover tightly with foil and bake for about 30 minutes or until the flesh collapses within the skin and has softened.

Remove carefully, and unwrap. Scoop out the flesh into a bowl, saving any juices. Discard the skins and the rosemary. Tip any reserved juices onto the flesh and mash together with a fork until smooth. Season well and add the lemon juice, cayenne or chilli. If liked, beat in a tablespoon of natural yogurt. Set aside to cool.

Meanwhile, make the melba toasts. Toast the pittas in a toaster, then split in two. Turn the oven heat down to 150°C, Gas Mark 3. Cut the pittas into triangles and place in the oven for 15 minutes or so until crisp and the edges have curled up slightly. Serve with small dollops of the aubergine salsa on top.

MAIN COURSES

Take the trouble to make at least one main course for yourself each day. Not only do main meals fill you up, but they also give you a good sense of well-being. After all, eating well and health-ily also includes enjoying your food.

MENU
Ratatouille and Rice
Golden Roots
Brazilian Stuffed Peppers
Thai Tofu Curry
Spinach and Quark Puff Bake
Tagine-style Vegetables and Harissa Couscous

RATATOUILLE AND RICE

Serves 2
Calories per portion/serving: 350
When I feel the need to cleanse my digestive system this is one of my favourite meals. In fact I make several portions at once and keep it on hand in the fridge ready for reheating. It fills me up and makes me feel so virtuous. Use brown or white basmati, Thai jasmine or Camargue red rice for this dish, not easy-cook.

INGREDIENTS
1 medium courgette
1 small red onion
1 small red or yellow pepper
1 small aubergine
2 fat cloves garlic, crushed
1 tablespoon olive oil
2 medium ripe tomatoes, chopped
sea salt and freshly ground black pepper
3 large fresh basil leaves, torn roughly
100g long-grain rice (see above)

TO SERVE
1 tablespoon sunflower seeds (optional)

METHOD
Chop the courgette, onion, pepper and aubergine into small, even chunks and place in a large saucepan with the garlic, olive

oil and 3 tablespoons water. Heat until the vegetables start to sizzle.

Clamp on the lid, lower the heat right down and cook for a good 10 minutes, shaking the pan occasionally without lifting the lid. (Chefs call this 'sweating' and it helps to cook vegetables in a small amount of oil. Good for flavour too.)

Add the tomatoes to the pan along with seasoning. Cover and cook for another 5 minutes or so, or until the tomatoes are mushy. Uncover and stir in the basil. Set aside to cool until just warm. (Ratatouille tastes much better warm, not too hot.)

Meanwhile, cook the rice according to the pack instructions. Remember that brown basmati and red rice take twice as long as white rice. Serve the vegetables on a bed of rice, scattered with the seeds.

GOLDEN ROOTS (WITH GREEN PASTA)

Serves 2–3
Calories per portion/serving: 110 (*or 225 with pasta*)
Now that modern transport has turned our seasonal food buying topsy turvy, it is possible to enjoy winter roots all year round. In summer you can buy baby roots with tender textures. Choose at least three root vegetables from the box opposite.

INGREDIENTS
your choice of at least 3 root vegetables (see box opposite)
1 leek, trimmed and sliced
200g tub fromage frais (0% fat for weight loss or 8% fat for weight maintenance)
freshly grated nutmeg, to taste
2 tablespoons chopped fresh parsley
sea salt and freshly ground black pepper

TO SERVE
Serve with green pasta and 1–2 teaspoons freshly grated parmesan

METHOD

Chop the roots into small even chunks. Place in a saucepan with the leek and barely cover with boiling water. Season with salt and simmer for 10 minutes or until just tender.

Meanwhile, cook the pasta according to the pack instructions.

Save a little of the water from the vegetables and drain the rest. Return the vegetables to the pan and chop with a knife to make a chunky purée. Stir in the fromage frais, nutmeg, parsley and seasoning to taste. For a softer texture, mix in some of the reserved vegetable water.

Drain the cooked pasta, stir in the vegetables and top with the parmesan. (When you have regained your sylph-like shape, you could even stir a small knob of butter into the vegetables – yum.)

Root vegetable alternatives
- 2 carrots, peeled thinly
- 1 large parsnip, peeled thinly
- 1 medium turnip or potato, peeled thinly
- 1/4 small swede, peeled
- 200g pumpkin flesh
- 200g squash, chopped

BRAZILIAN STUFFED PEPPERS
....

Serves 2

Calories per portion/serving: 230

Add an exotic touch to a familiar supper favourite. Good served with Carrot, Mint and Cheese Salad (page 125).

INGREDIENTS
1 yellow pepper
1 red pepper
1 onion, chopped
2 fat cloves garlic, crushed
1–2 large fresh green chillies, deseeded and chopped

1 teaspoon olive oil
1 teaspoon ground coriander
$^{1}/_{4}$ teaspoon cumin seeds
good pinch ground cinnamon
good pinch dried thyme
200g can red kidney beans, drained and rinsed
1 slice wholemeal or granary bread
sea salt and freshly ground black pepper

METHOD

Halve the peppers lengthways, remove the seeds and ribs but leave the stalks on. Preheat a grill until hot and cook the peppers on both sides until they start to soften, about 7 minutes. Remove and cool.

Now for the filling. Put the onion, garlic and chillies into a saucepan with the oil and 2 tablespoons water. Heat until they start to sizzle, then cover and turn the heat right down. Cook for 10 minutes, shaking the pan occasionally, but don't lift the lid. Uncover and stir in the spices and thyme, cooking for a few seconds. Remove from the heat.

Mash the beans slightly with a fork. Rub the bread on a coarse grater or pass through a food processor to make crumbs. Stir both into the onion mix and season well.

Spoon into the pepper shells and brown under the grill for a few minutes to crisp the top slightly.

THAI TOFU CURRY
· ·

Serves 2
Calories per portion/serving: 360
Thai 'green' curries need no pre-frying, yet still taste rich and delicious. For the traditional coconut flavour without too many extra calories, make a light 'stock' using desiccated coconut. Choose smoked or marinated tofu for the best flavour (usually found in chilled cabinets, near the cheese). Classic Thai ingredients are available from larger supermarkets or local Oriental food stores.

INGREDIENTS

1 tablespoon desiccated coconut
300ml vegetable stock made from
    boiling water and stock powder
1 medium onion, chopped roughly
1 fat clove garlic, crushed
1 large fresh green chilli, seeded and
    sliced thinly
2 tablespoons light soy sauce
sea salt
200g smoked or marinated tofu
1 fresh red chilli, sliced into thin rings (optional)
100g Thai jasmine rice or Thai rice noodles
2–3 large fresh basil leaves, torn
2–3 sprigs fresh coriander

Thai 'green' curries need no pre-frying, yet still taste rich and delicious.

TO SERVE

sesame seeds (optional)

METHOD

Steep the coconut in the just-boiled stock for 30 minutes, then drain, reserving the liquid and discarding the coconut. Meanwhile, blend the onion, garlic and green chilli to a purée in a food processor.

Place in a saucepan with the coconut liquid, the sauces and a little salt. Bring to the boil, then simmer for 2 minutes.

Cut the tofu into small cubes and plop into the sauce along with the red chilli strips, if using. Return to a simmer and cook for another 2 minutes. Meanwhile, cook the rice or noodles according to the pack instructions.

Stir the fresh herbs into the curry and reheat if liked. Serve with the rice or noodles. A light sprinkling of sesame seeds will add an attractive touch.

SPINACH AND QUARK PUFF BAKE

Serves 2
Calories per portion/serving: 300
Quark, a soft cheese made from skimmed milk, is normally associated with cheesecakes, but it also makes a good creamy base for light, fluffy, vegetable bakes. For a stronger cheesy flavour, use fresh parmesan.

INGREDIENTS

200g bag young spinach leaves
2 salad onions, chopped finely
200g tub quark
1 tablespoon light soy sauce
2 large free-range eggs, separated
2 teaspoons freshly grated parmesan cheese
sea salt and freshly ground black pepper
low-fat cooking spray
1 tablespoon dried breadcrumbs

METHOD

Cook the spinach according to the instructions on the bag. (The best way is in the microwave.) Drain and cool, squeezing out excess water using the back of a ladle or a wooden spoon, then chop finely.

Mix with the chopped onions, quark, soy sauce, egg yolks, parmesan cheese and seasoning.

Preheat the oven to 190°C, Gas Mark 5. Lightly spray a 1-litre ovenproof dish or soufflé dish with a little of the cooking spray and shake the breadcrumbs around the sides. (This helps the mixture rise up more evenly.)

Whisk the egg whites to the soft peak stage in a large grease-free bowl, using a balloon or electric rotary whisk, then carefully fold into the spinach mixture using a large metal spoon.

Scoop into the prepared dish, levelling the top. Bake for 30 minutes or so until risen and very slightly wobbly. Eat instantly.

TAGINE-STYLE VEGETABLES WITH HARISSA COUSCOUS

Serves 2

Calories per portion/serving: 375

Tagines are traditional Moroccan conical earthenware dishes used for the gentle cooking of spicy stews, the idea being that steam collects at the top of the cone and gently moistens the simmering stew underneath. We use the same romantic notion for winter vegetables but an everyday saucepan with a domed lid will do. The hot and spicy harissa paste is sold in a tube (available from large supermarkets).

INGREDIENTS

1 large carrot, chopped in chunks
1 large parsnip, chopped in chunks
1 red onion, sliced thinly
1 green pepper, cored and sliced
2 fat cloves garlic, chopped
$1/4$ teaspoon ground cumin
1 teaspoon ground coriander
$1/4$ teaspoon ground cinnamon
1 bay leaf
200ml vegetable stock
200ml tomato juice
sea salt and freshly ground pepper
1 tablespoon fresh lemon juice
1 medium courgette, sliced
150g easy-to-cook couscous
harissa paste, to taste

TO SERVE

chopped fresh coriander or parsley

METHOD

Put all the vegetables, with the exception of the courgette, into a saucepan with the garlic, spices, bay leaf, stock and tomato juice. Add seasoning. Bring to the boil, stirring, then cover and simmer very, very gently for 10–12 minutes, stirring once or twice.

Add the lemon juice and courgette, and cook uncovered for another 5 minutes.

Meanwhile, prepare the couscous according to the pack instructions, but make sure it is not too wet. It helps to stir the grains with a fork as they absorb the water. Season well, then stir in harissa paste to taste. Add a cautious amount at first, as it can knock your socks off.

Check the vegetable 'stew' for seasoning, then serve with the couscous, sprinkled with chopped fresh herbs.

LENTIL 'BOLOGNESE' WITH GRILLED VEGETABLES AND PASTA

Serves 4
Calories per portion/serving: 270
The humble red lentil is the lean veggie's lifeline. It is high in protein and fibre, tasty, fat free and best of all – it is a fast thickener. A few tablespoons sprinkled into a simmering stew will produce a good all-purpose sauce in under 20 minutes, great for pasta or baby new potatoes. It freezes if you have any left; or can be kept chilled for up to 3 days.

A serving hint: instead of grated cheese, sprinkle over a coarsely grated carrot. If on a weight maintenance diet, 1–2 teaspoons freshly grated parmesan are allowable.

INGREDIENTS
1 onion, chopped
2 fat cloves garlic, crushed
1 large fresh red chilli, seeded and chopped (optional)
2 teaspoons olive oil
about 4 tablespoons dry white wine (optional but nice)
420g can chopped tomatoes
150ml vegetable stock or water
5 tablespoons split red lentils
$^1/_2$ teaspoon dried oregano

sea salt and freshly ground
    black pepper
200g pasta shapes
1 large red or yellow pepper,
    quartered and cored
2 medium courgettes, quar-
    tered lengthways
low-fat cooking spray

The humble red lentil is the lean veggie's lifeline. It is high in protein and fibre, tasty and fat free.

METHOD

Put the onion, garlic and chilli, if using, into a saucepan and vigorously stir in the oil so that everything is well coated. Add 2 tablespoons water, heat to a sizzle, then turn the heat right down, cover and cook for 5 minutes, shaking the pan once or twice.

Remember: 'wet' pasta doesn't need lots of fattening butter or oil.

Uncover, add the wine (if using) and cook until it evaporates. Stir in the tomatoes, stock or water, lentils, oregano and seasoning. Bring to the boil, then simmer, uncovered, for about 15 minutes, stirring occasionally. Check the seasoning and set aside.

Meanwhile, heat the grill until very hot. Lay the pepper and courgette slices on the grid and spray with low-fat cooking spray. Cook for about 5 minutes or until lightly charred. Then turn and cook the other sides. Season, remove and cool.

Cook the pasta according to the pack instructions. Drain, but don't shake dry, and tip it straight into a serving dish. (Remember: 'wet' pasta doesn't need lots of fattening butter or oil.) Serve with the lentil sauce and the grilled vegetables.

SQUASH AND BROAD BEANS WITH ORANGE GINGER SOY SAUCE

Serves 2
Calories per portion/serving: 210

Squashes come in all sorts of tempting colours and shapes, and they store for weeks. A heavy blow with a sharp knife cleaves them in half for easier peeling and chopping. They are teamed here in an Oriental-style sauce with high-protein baby broad beans (easy to find in supermarket freezer cabinets). This dish is good with a little rice or pasta.

INGREDIENTS

1 medium-size squash (e.g. acorn, butternut)
1 teaspoon lower-fat olive oil spread
1 onion, sliced thinly
1 fat clove garlic, crushed
200g frozen broad beans, thawed
pinch dried sage
sea salt and freshly ground black pepper
juice of 1 small orange
1 tablespoon light soy sauce
1 teaspoon ginger purée (available in tubes and small jars)
tiny trickle roasted sesame oil

TO SERVE

1 grissini Italian garlic or sesame breadstick, roughly crushed

METHOD

Peel and seed the squash, then chop into small chunks. Boil in lightly salted water, to just cover, for 5–7 minutes until just tender. Drain.

Meanwhile, melt the olive oil spread in a small saucepan with 2 tablespoons water and cook the onion and garlic gently for 5 minutes until softened.

Add the beans, sage and seasoning. (If you have time, pop the beans from their pods first.) Cook for about 3 minutes, then add the orange juice, soy sauce, ginger and sesame. Boil for 2 minutes, then stir in the squash and seasoning.

Reheat until bubbling and delicious and serve topped with the breadstick crumbs.

OH SO SIMPLE SPAGHETTI AND MUSHROOMS

••

Serves 2

Calories per portion/serving: 275

I feel so worthy eating wholewheat spaghetti, especially as there are some pasta sauces that complement it well. One of these is a quick and easy, hit-the-pan mushroom medley. Sometimes you can buy 'gourmet selections' of different mushrooms, otherwise organic chestnut brown mushrooms are good plate fellows.

INGREDIENTS

150–200g wholewheat spaghetti (depending on your diet level)
1 teaspoon extra-virgin olive oil
small handful fresh parsley sprigs, scissor-snipped (see box, overleaf)

SAUCE

200g mushrooms, any variety, or a mixture, sliced thinly
2 fat cloves garlic, crushed
150ml vegetable stock made with stock powder
little splash of dry vermouth, white wine or dry sherry
sea salt and freshly ground black pepper
2 tablespoons half-fat crème fraiche or 0% fat fromage frais (depending on your diet level)

METHOD

Boil the spaghetti according to the pack instructions. Because it is wholewheat, it will take longer than normal, so you can make the sauce in the meantime.

Put the mushrooms, garlic, stock and vermouth, wine or sherry in a saucepan, bring to the boil, then lower the heat to a simmer and cook for 3–5 minutes, stirring occasionally until softened.

Season well, then remove from the heat. Stir in the crème fraiche or fromage frais and set aside.

By now the spaghetti should be ready. Drain, return to the pan and toss in the oil and parsley. Serve straight away with the sauce.

To chop fresh parsley or other herbs quickly, pop a few sprigs into a mug or small jug and snip several times with scissors.

RISOTTO TO SUIT

Serves 2
Calories per portion/serving: 320

Once you can make a basic risotto, the world's your culinary oyster. There are so many ways that you can vary the additional flavourings to create a new dish each time. So here is a simple basic recipe with some suggested variations to make it more of a meal. Choose one from the box opposite.

However, you do need proper risotto rice (e.g. Arborio, Carnaroli or Vialone Nano) to make the dish creamy, with a good al dente bite to the grain.

INGREDIENTS

1 litre vegetable stock, ideally fresh (see page 69) or made with
   good stock powder
1 onion, chopped
1 fat clove garlic, crushed
2 teaspoons olive oil
150g risotto rice
2 tablespoons dry vermouth or 3 tablespoons dry white wine
1 tablespoon freshly grated parmesan cheese
sea salt and freshly ground black pepper

METHOD

First prepare the ingredients for your chosen variation below and set aside. Make sure the stock has just boiled and keep it hot.

Put the onion and garlic in a large saucepan with the oil and 2 table-spoons water. Heat until sizzling and cook on a gentle heat for 5 minutes until softened.

> *Once you can make a basic risotto, the world's your culinary oyster.*

Stir in the rice and cook for 2 minutes, then add the vermouth or wine and cook until it evaporates away.

Stir in a quarter of the hot stock. Cook on a medium simmer, stirring frequently until the liquid is all absorbed.

Add another quarter of the remaining stock and cook, again stirring, until it is absorbed. Continue like this until the stock is all used and the rice is creamy, plump and tender. This should take about 15–18 minutes. If the rice needs extra liquid, simply add boiling water from a kettle in small amounts, again stirring it in. Season well and stir in the parmesan.

Now, mix in your chosen addition and cook for an extra 2 minutes to reheat. Serve immediately before the risotto loses its creamy texture.

Variations

Choose one of the following:

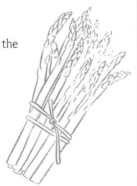

- **Asparagus** – peel and chop the stems of 150g fresh asparagus, reserving the tips. Blanch the stems in boiling water, drain, then mix with the tips and the grated zest of 1 lemon.

- **Mushroom** – soak 20g dried cep (porcini) mushrooms in boiling water to just cover. Use the liquor in the risotto stock.
- **Primavera vegetables** – chop a 150g selection of baby sweetcorn, carrots, green beans and peas. Blanch for 2 minutes in boiling water and drain.
- **Beetroot and mushroom** – chop 100g unvinegared cooked beets in small cubes. Slice 100g button mushrooms and cook in a little stock.

LASAGNE ROLLS OR EASY CANNELLONI

Serves 2
Calories per portion/serving: 417
Ordinary lasagne is messy to eat and tubes of cannelloni are fussy to fill. So, here's a good compromise – lasagne pasta rolled round a chunky vegetable filling. Top with half-fat crème fraiche instead of a fattening sauce and serve with a crisp green salad.

INGREDIENTS
4 sheets lasagne pasta
1 onion, chopped
1 fat clove garlic, crushed
1 stick celery, chopped finely
1 carrot, coarsely grated
4 large button mushrooms
1 tablespoon olive oil
good pinch dried oregano
200g can chopped tomatoes
1 tablespoon tomato purée
1 teaspoon pesto sauce (optional)
sea salt and freshly ground black pepper
2 tablespoons half-fat crème fraiche
1 Italian grissini breadstick, crushed

METHOD

Blanch the lasagne pasta in a large pan of boiling water for 5 minutes, then drain and keep in a bowl of cold water. Preheat the oven to 190°C, Gas Mark 5.

Put the onion, garlic, celery, carrot and mushrooms into a saucepan with the oil and 2 tablespoons water. Heat to a sizzle, then cover and cook on a low heat for 5 minutes until softened.

Uncover, add the oregano, tomatoes, purée and pesto, if using. Season well and bring to the boil, then simmer uncovered for 5–10 minutes or until the liquid has evaporated a little to reduce.

Drain the lasagne sheets and pat dry with kitchen paper towel. Divide the filling between the sheets and roll up. Place join-side down in a shallow ovenproof dish, then spoon on the crème fraiche and top with the crushed breadstick. Bake in the preheated oven for 15 minutes or until piping hot.

PENNE PUTTANESCA

Serves 2
Calories per portion/serving: 405

A spicy classic once popular with Roman ladies of the night but now happily eaten in the most respectable homes! To make it more of a meal, stir in some canned borlotti beans. Use large fresh red chillies for a milder flavour, or small bird's-eye ones for a fiery punch.

INGREDIENTS

1 onion, chopped
2 fat cloves garlic, crushed
1 large fresh red chilli, seeded and sliced, or 1–2 small red chillies, chopped
2 teaspoons olive oil
200g can chopped tomatoes
few shakes mushroom ketchup or light soy sauce
$^1/_2$ teaspoon dried Italian mixed herbs or herbes de Provence
sea salt and freshly ground black pepper

1 tablespoon chopped pitted black olives
150g penne pasta

TO SERVE
scissor-snipped fresh parsley or basil
3 tablespoons canned borlotti beans, drained and rinsed (optional)

METHOD
Put the onion, garlic and chilli into a saucepan with the oil and
2 tablespoons water. Bring to a sizzle, then turn the heat down
to low. Cover and cook for 5 minutes until softened.

Uncover, add the tomatoes, mushroom ketchup or soy sauce,
herbs and seasoning. Simmer for a further 5 minutes, then mix
in the olives.

Meanwhile, cook the pasta according to the pack instructions. Drain and mix into the sauce along with the snipped fresh
herbs. Add the beans, if using, and reheat for 1–2 minutes. Eat hot.

VEGETABLE ROASTIES WITH PAPRIKA YOGURT SAUCE

Serves 2
Calories per portion/serving: 225
It is possible to achieve a roast vegetable flavour by using a very
small amount of oil if you cook at a high oven temperature. The
secret is to rub the wedges of root vegetables with the
measured oil in a food bag so that they are evenly and lightly
coated. A creamy low-fat spicy sauce accompanies. Serve with
lightly cooked cabbage, Brussels sprouts or beans.

INGREDIENTS
1 medium-size baking potato (about 150g)
1 large carrot or medium sweet potato
1 large parsnip
2 teaspoons olive oil
1–2 good pinches dried thyme or mixed herbs
sea salt and freshly ground black pepper

SAUCE

150g tub low-fat 'bio' natural
    yogurt
1 tablespoon mild or sweet chilli
    sauce or few drops hot pepper
    sauce
1 teaspoon paprika
1/2 teaspoon ground cumin
1/2 teaspoon garlic salt or 1 clove
    garlic, crushed
1/2 teaspoon dried oregano

It is possible to achieve a roast vegetable flavour by using a very small amount of oil if you cook at a high oven temperature.

TO SERVE

chopped fresh parsley or chives

METHOD

Preheat the oven to 220°C, Gas Mark 7, and place a non-stick baking sheet near the top of the oven. Heat for a good 10 minutes.

Meanwhile, prepare the vegetables. Cut them into even-size wedges no more than 2cm thick. Pop them into a large poly food bag with the oil. Seal the bag with a twist tie and rub everything together well for 1–2 minutes so that all the edges are coated in oil.

When the oven is good and hot, carefully remove the hot tray. Tip out the vegetable wedges and spread in a single layer on the tray. Sprinkle over the thyme or mixed herbs and season well.

Return the tray to the oven and cook for 15–20 minutes, without stirring, until the edges are nicely browned, the potato wedges have puffed a little and the flesh is just tender.

Meanwhile, make the sauce by simply mixing everything together. Season well. Tip the roasties out on a serving plate, sprinkle with chopped herbs and serve the sauce alongside in a bowl.

'STIR-STEAM' OF VEGETABLES

Serves 2
Calories per portion/serving: 180
Stir-frying can be quite a high-fat method of cooking. So, I

developed a way of cooking vegetables to a similar level of crunch, using either a steamer or the microwave oven. They still have the same tasty aroma but much less fat. Marvellously low in calories yet high in satisfaction. You might like to flavour the water for steaming with a stem of fresh lemon grass, one or two star anise, a few strips of root ginger and a crushed bulb of garlic.

Serve with steaming rice noodles or a small bowl of lightly sticky Thai rice. For extra protein, add a few cubes of smoked or marinated tofu.

INGREDIENTS
250g selection of crisp Oriental style-vegetables (choose 3 or 4 from the box opposite)
2 salad onions, sliced diagonally into chunks
sea salt and freshly ground black pepper
2 tablespoons light soy sauce
1 teaspoon roasted sesame oil

TO SERVE
1–2 tablespoons chopped fresh coriander or parsley
few pinches toasted sesame seeds

METHOD
Prepare your choice of vegetables so that they are all about the same size.

If steaming, put a pan of water on to boil. Place the vegetables (including the salad onions) in a steamer basket over the simmering water, season, then cover and steam for about 5 minutes.

If using a microwave oven, place the vegetables in a non-metallic bowl with 3 tablespoons of water and seasoning. Cover, venting the side a little, and cook on full power for 3 minutes. Uncover, stir well, re-cover and cook for another 2 minutes. Allow to stand for 1 minute or so and drain.

When the vegetables are ready, place in a warm serving bowl and toss with the soy sauce and sesame oil. Sprinkle with the herbs and sesame seeds and serve immediately.

> **Oriental-style vegetables**
> Choose 3–4 of the following:
> - baby sweetcorns
> - mangetout
> - strips of red pepper
> - Chinese cabbage or pak choi
> - baby carrots
> - asparagus tips
> - oyster mushrooms

SALADS

A good-sized salad daily will help you easily achieve the goal of eating five fruits and vegetables a day. If you keep the dressings low in fat, salads will also help you lose weight or maintain your ideal weight.

The problem with many salads is that they can be high in oil-rich dressings or include high-fat ingredients, such as grated cheese and nuts. Remember: the word 'salad' is not another name for a low-calorie dish.

And don't serve salads too cold. Chilling can affect flavour, so if you make and chill a salad ahead, let it return to room temperature 30 minutes or so before you tuck in.

FIVE SALAD BOWLS – WITH DRESSINGS AND FLOURISHES

MENU
Indonesian Rice and Egg-strip Salad
Carrot, Mint and Cheese Salad
Beetroot with Horseradish Dressing
Fatoush
Caesar's Salad with Oven-crisp Croutons

A good-sized salad daily will help you easily achieve the goal of eating five fruits and vegetables a day.

Serves 2

Calories per portion/serving: 385

This combination of hot brown basmati rice tossed into chopped and chilled vegetables makes a spicy and thoroughly modern fusion-food salad. Top with strips of flat omelette to turn it into a main meal, although this can be omitted if you want to cut down on calories.

INGREDIENTS

100g brown basmati rice

1 large free-range egg (optional)

1 teaspoon light soy sauce (optional)

low-fat cooking spray

2 salad onions, chopped

125g beansprouts, preferably a mixture (see home-sprouted sprouts, page 85)

1 tender celery stick, sliced thinly

$1/2$ small red pepper, cored and cut in thin strips

2 slices canned pineapple in natural juice, patted dry and chopped

2 tablespoons chopped fresh coriander

DRESSING

1 teaspoon sesame seed oil

juice of 1 lime

1 fat clove garlic, crushed

$1/4 - 1/2$ teaspoon hot chilli powder (or few drops hot pepper sauce)

1 tablespoon light soy sauce

1 teaspoon clear honey

1 tablespoon rice wine vinegar

freshly ground black pepper

TO SERVE

1 teaspoon toasted sesame seeds

METHOD

First, make the dressing by shaking everything together in a screw-topped jar. Set aside.

   Put the brown basmati on to cook, following the pack instructions. Drain in a colander and set aside.

Now if wished, make the omelette: heat a small non-stick frying pan until you can feel a good steady heat rising. Beat the egg with the soy sauce plus a little pepper. Spray the pan lightly with the cooking spray, then pour in the egg. Cook on a low heat, without stirring or tipping, until all the runny egg has set. Flip over briefly, then slide out onto kitchen paper towel and pat dry of oil. Cut the omelette into thin strips.

Mix all the prepared vegetables and pineapple in a big bowl and toss in the dressing. Mix in the chopped herbs, then stir in the hot rice. Season and mix well. Serve on flat plates garnished with the egg strips, if using, and sprinkled with sesame seeds.

CARROT, MINT AND CHEESE SALAD
....

Serves 1
Calories per portion/serving: 120
A nice simple lunch-bowl salad. Use a half-fat hard cheese or, for an even lower-calorie dish, a tub of low-fat cottage cheese.

INGREDIENTS
2 medium carrots
1 salad onion, chopped
1 tablespoon sunflower seeds
1 tablespoon chopped fresh mint
juice of $1/2$ lemon
sea salt and freshly ground black pepper
25g half-fat Cheddar or a small tub of low-fat cottage cheese

TO SERVE
rocket leaves (optional)

METHOD
Coarsely grate the carrots, then mix with the onion, seeds and mint. Toss with the lemon juice and season well. Set aside for 10 minutes to let the flavours mellow.

Cut the hard cheese (if using) into small cubes. Mix the cheese of your choice into the carrot salad. Serve as it is or on a bed of rocket leaves.

BEETROOT IN HORSERADISH DRESSING

Serves 2
Calories per portion/serving: 190

We really should follow our European neighbours and eat more beetroot! It is so delicious, especially when not served swimming in sharp vinegary dressing. To make this salad more of a main meal, serve with quartered hard-boiled eggs.

INGREDIENTS

300g cooked baby beetroots, not in vinegar dressing
1 salad onion, chopped, or 1 tablespoon chopped fresh chives
3 tablespoons low-fat 'bio' natural yogurt
1 teaspoon horseradish relish
sea salt and freshly ground black pepper

TO SERVE

1 punnet mustard and cress

METHOD

Chop the beets into small dice, then mix with the onions or chives. Stir the yogurt and horseradish together with the seasoning and mix in the beets. Snip the cress over the top to serve.

FATOUSH

Serves 2
Calories per portion/serving: 245

A popular Egyptian dish of chopped salad vegetables and soaked country bread. Make this a few hours ahead so that the flavours seep into each other. The optional sumac is an astringent ground herb used in many parts of the Eastern Mediterranean. You can find it in halal shops and some Middle Eastern delis.

INGREDIENTS

100g country-style crusty bread, or baguette
2 ripe tomatoes, chopped small
¹/₃ cucumber, chopped small
about 4 large radishes, chopped

1 small onion, grated
1–2 fat cloves garlic, crushed
1 little gem lettuce, shredded
small handful fresh mint leaves, chopped
sea salt and freshly ground black pepper
2 tablespoons lemon juice
2 teaspoons olive oil

TO SERVE
2 teaspoons sumac (optional)

METHOD
Break the bread into small chunks and place in a large salad bowl. Sprinkle with cold water until it is lightly soaked.

Put all the chopped vegetables, garlic, lettuce and mint leaves on top, seasoning well in between. Cover and chill for 1–2 hours.

Mix the lemon juice and olive oil together and sprinkle over. Using two large spoons, toss everything together in the bowl. Sprinkle with the sumac, if using, just before serving.

CAESAR'S SALAD WITH OVEN-CRISP CROUTONS

Serves 2
Calories per portion/serving: 155

In the 1930s, an Italian American, Caesar Cardini, created this timeless salad, which is now popular the world over. The original required a rich egg and anchovy dressing plus deep-fried croutons. There is no need to miss this out completely though – bake a batch of lower-fat croutons in the oven and store in an airtight jar to sprinkle over crisp leaves whenever you feel like a crunch. Add extra salad vegetables if you want to make it more of a meal, such as grated carrot, cucumber or sliced radishes.

INGREDIENTS
1 romaine or small cos lettuce
sea salt and freshly ground black pepper

DRESSING

2 teaspoons extra-virgin olive oil
2 teaspoons white wine vinegar
2 teaspoons freshly grated parmesan cheese

CROUTONS

2 slices thick white or brown (e.g. granary) bread
low-fat olive oil cooking spray
good pinch dried oregano
good few pinches garlic salt

TO SERVE

1 tablespoon fresh chopped parsley or chives or both

METHOD

Tear the leaves into bite-sized pieces. If necessary, wash and spin them. Place in a bowl, season with salt and plenty of pepper, then cover and chill for at least 1 hour to crisp.

In a cup mix together the oil, vinegar and parmesan.

Meanwhile, make the croutons. Cut the bread into small 1–2 cm cubes. Preheat the oven to 180°C, Gas Mark 4. Spread the bread cubes in a single layer on a baking sheet, spray lightly and evenly with the olive oil spray and sprinkle with oregano and garlic salt.

Bake for 20 minutes, turning once, until light golden brown. Remove and allow to cool, when they will crisp up. Use half for this salad and store the remainder in an air-tight food container.

To serve, toss the dressing into the chilled leaves with the chopped herbs and scatter over the croutons.

LOW-FAT DRESSINGS

As we know, oils and fats have 9 calories per gram, which means that every tablespoon contains up to around 120 calories. Which is fine if you are making a dressing that will be divided between three or four people, but not if you are eating it alone.

The normal rule of thumb when calculating dressings is one-third vinegar to two-thirds oil. Put like that, it is easy to see how an apparently innocuous salad of virtually zero-calorie leaves and vegetables can end up dripping in calories once it's been drenched with dressing.

But it is possible to have some delicious alternatives with much lower dressings!

Try these:

- Toss leaves or coarsely grated vegetables with the juice of 1 fresh lemon or lime plus sea salt and freshly ground black pepper.
- Tomatoes and cucumber make their own juices simply by being sprinkled fairly lightly with sea salt and left in a colander or bowl. This is known by chefs as degorging. These juices can make a light natural dressing in themselves. (Wash the salt off the vegetables after degorging.)
- Ready-seasoned Japanese rice wine vinegar (also known as sushi dressing) makes a delicious dressing for hot rice, pasta and potatoes – with zilch calories.
- Grate a quarter of a cucumber and 1 small onion into a bowl and sprinkle with 1 teaspoon salt. Leave to degorge for 15 minutes, then mix in 3 tablespoons low-fat yogurt or silken tofu, and 1 tablespoon chopped fresh mint and/or parsley. Use instead of mayonnaise.
- Put 2 tablespoons apple juice, 1 tablespoon white wine or rice wine, 2 teaspoons light soy sauce and 1 teaspoon clear honey in a screw-topped jar with 1 crushed clove of garlic,

> *Ready-seasoned Japanese rice wine vinegar makes a delicious dressing for hot rice, pasta and potatoes – with zilch calories.*

freshly ground black pepper and some sea salt. Shake well to mix. Alternatively, use fresh orange juice instead of apple, basalmic vinegar instead of wine vinegar and coarse-grained mustard in place of the soy sauce.

SWEET AND HAPPY ENDINGS

Whether you are a vegetarian or a meat eater, puddings and desserts can be a problem when you are trying to lose weight. But there's no reason to deprive yourself of treats all the time. After all, there's a limit to how many apples and oranges you can eat in a day!

Remember, **fats** are one of the main culprits for weight gain, so keep your intake of creamy foods to a bare minimum and watch the sugars.

A *little* ordinary **sugar**, or fruit sugar such as fructose which is found in honey, will do you no harm.

Nuts, though, are high in calories – anything up to 600 calories per 100g. But if you toast and chop a few, you may find that 1 teaspoon of chopped toasted almonds or pecans goes a long way when sprinkled over sliced fruits, yogurts, etc.

Chocolate is definitely one food to watch because of the fat and sugar. But, if you choose a chocolate with a high percentage of cocoa solids (60% plus) you will have a stronger flavour with less fat and can restrict yourself to 1–2 squares when the longing for a chocoholic fix takes hold. One tip I find useful is to finely grate a couple of squares of high-quality chocolate and store it in the fridge, ready to sprinkle lightly over yogurt, fromage frais or fruits.

The following recipe is for a good chocolate dipping sauce. Although not exactly strict diet fare, it is fine for an occasional treat, surrounded by a plate of fresh strawberries, cherries or chunks of fresh pineapple.

> *A little ordinary sugar, or fruit sugar such as fructose which is found in honey, will do you no harm.*

CHOCOLATE DIPPING SAUCE

Serves 3–4
Calories per portion/serving: 75 ⌣ (300 for full amount)
Make sure the chocolate is at least 60% cocoa solids.

INGREDIENTS
50g good-quality dark chocolate
1 teaspoon clear honey
ground cinnamon (optional)

METHOD
Break the chocolate into a heatproof bowl. Add 100ml water and the honey. Heat, either in the microwave on full power for 2 minutes, stirring once only, or over a pan of gently simmering water. Do not overheat before stirring or the chocolate will seize up. Add a dusting of ground cinnamon, if using. Cool (it thickens on cooling) and stir before serving.

FRUIT SALADS

Try to eat a bowl of at least three fruits each day. Make one of them a **juicy fruit**, like an orange, pineapple, melon or mango; then you won't have to worry about the calories in high-sugar syrup.

A good tip is to choose only **ripe fruits**. This will help cut down on sugar, although if you do need an extra sweet boost, sprinkle over a pinch or two of powdered artificial sweetener. Don't heat these sweeteners or they will taste bitter. If you like stewed fruit, poach them first in a little water or apple juice and only add the sweetener when they have cooled down.

My favourite natural sweetener is a trickle of **maple syrup** –

> *Putting together a fruit salad is also an excellent way of trying out an exotic fruit variety that is new to you to see if you like it.*

and because it is quite light and runny, a little goes a long way.

I also sometimes sprinkle fruits with **icing sugar**, although weight for weight it has the same calorific value as ordinary sugar. However, it tastes sweeter than ordinary sugar because it dissolves more quickly on the tongue.

Another way of adding flavour is to use **flower waters** – rose or orange blossom are particularly good.

Putting together a **fruit salad** is also an excellent way of trying out an exotic fruit variety that is new to you to see if you like it. I am now particularly fond of Asian pears and mangosteens. One or two of these popped into my supermarket basket have now replaced a chocolate bar as a treat.

Dried Fruits

These are excellent sources of minerals and fibre, but if you gorge on too many, the calories mount up. There are excellent supplies of ready-to-eat dried fruits such as plump raisins, apricots, figs and prunes (*do* try the French pruneaux d'Agen – divine) but keep a lookout too for dried mangoes, peaches, cherries, cranberries and blueberries.

Take care that you buy dried fruits, not candied fruits, which are dripping in sugar syrup.

Organic dried fruits have an extra-special flavour but I do have unpleasant memories of the after-effects of a surfeit of fragrant hunza apricots. As I said, they are excellent sources of dietary fibre!

DAIRY PRODUCTS AND MILKY PUDS

These are, of course, high in calcium. But in order for your body to utilize this vital mineral, you do need a good intake of vitamin C.

It seems that there are now more low-fat dairy goods on the

shelves than normal-fat, so you will have a lot of choice. And low- or no-fat doesn't have to mean very sharp or acidic flavours. **Yogurts**, for instance – the mild culture 'bio' yogurts taste lightly creamy. Sweeten, if you like, with artificial sweetener (unless they are already sweetened) or trickle in 1–2 teaspoons of flower honey or, my favourite, unrefined light muscovado sugar.

I love **rice puddings** made with skimmed milk, not rich creamy milk (the starch makes them creamy without fat) and cooked on top of the stove using a fragrant rice such as Thai jasmine or basmati. My favourite recipe, below, uses one of two elegant rices: Thai jasmine or basmati.

RICE PUDDING

Serves 4

Calories per portion/serving: 144

Nice with a little fat-free fromage frais or half-fat crème fraiche stirred in, plus a dusting of ground cinnamon. Good too as a sundae spooned over sliced red berry fruits, peaches or bananas.

INGREDIENTS

100g Thai jasmine or basmati rice
600ml skimmed milk
3–4 cardamom pods
1 stem lemon grass, 1 bay leaf or 1 stick cinnamon
artificial sweetener, unrefined sugar or honey

METHOD

In a saucepan, combine the rice with the skimmed milk and the cardamom pods, plus the lemon grass, bay leaf or cinnamon. Simmer for about 20 minutes until reduced down and creamy, stirring often. Cool and sweeten with artificial sweetener, unrefined sugar or honey. Remove the whole flavourings before serving.

CHAPTER EIGHT

Menu Planning

Combinations of meals are very personal. When planning menus for other people, we tend to assume that they like all foods. But we also have to take into account whether or not the diet is nutritionally balanced.

Instead of worrying about each meal, think in terms of broad outlines. Each meal should have a good base of complex **carbohydrates** – bread, rice, pasta or potato. Add to this one or two pieces of **fruit** or a couple of **vegetables**. Then include a tablespoon or so of a **protein** food, such as pulses, yogurt or tofu; maybe an egg or even a small amount of cheese or a little fistful of nuts or seeds. You'll find that extras like **fats or oils and sugars** will appear automatically along the way, which is fine as long as they are in modest moderation.

So if you plan to cook one of the main meals in this book, look at the balance of ingredients and see what you can add. Would a chunk of crusty wholegrain bread be a good accompaniment, or what about a bowl of rice or a baked potato zapped quickly in the microwave? Starters and sweet things you can keep as basic as you like or have a simple light main course with a more elaborate milky or fruity pud at the end.

Here are seven ideas for each meal occasion during the day. You put them together as you like.

On page 138 you will find ideas for beating a snack attack.

BREAKFASTS

- Bowl of microwave porridge (page 90) with a piece of fresh fruit or a glass of fresh juice, 1 apple or orange.
- 2 slices wholegrain toast with 2 scant teaspoons low-fat vegetable spread, Marmite, honey or high-fruit jam. Or instead of vegetable spread, use a thin scraping of peanut

butter. Small mug or teacup of low-fat hot chocolate with skimmed milk.

- Bowl of wholewheat, sugar-free cereal topped with a sliced peach, apricot or banana, plus skimmed milk. Try mixing two cereals together such as crispy rice and All-Bran or Bran Flakes and Shredded Wheat.
- Tub low-fat live yogurt with chopped fresh fruits, a teaspoon of wheatgerm or bran sprinkled with ground cinnamon and a trickle of honey or maple syrup.
- Wholemeal muffin, split and toasted and spread thinly with low-fat soft cheese, a teaspoon of honey and topped with a small sliced banana.
- Juicy fruit bowl – simply mix together a selection of sliced or chopped fruits. Some could be canned in natural juice and drained as a base, such as pineapple chunks or apricots. Add a sliced crisp apple or peach, some melon, a kiwi or a small sliced banana, and snip over 2–3 stoned no-need-to-soak prunes. It's amazing how filling a bowl of fruit can be. Use at least three fruits, ideally four.
- Cooked breakfast – choose scrambled eggs on toast (see page 92), poached eggs, or try Squashy Tomatoes on Pesto Toast (page 94). Also nice are halved button mushrooms (allow about 100g a head), cooked in a little seasoned water until just soft, then drained and tossed with a shake of light soy sauce and 1–2 teaspoons light crème fraiche, nestled on a slice of wholemeal toast.

LUNCH

Keep this light.
- Any big soup from pages 98–101, accompanied by 1 slice of crusty bread or 3 rye crispbreads. Some crisp vegetables or a piece of fruit.
- Medium/small baked potato with Carrot, Mint and Cheese Salad (page 125).
- Chickpea and Greek Salad Pitta (page 96).
- Chunk of French bread (about 10cm length) spread lightly

with low-fat soft cheese or half-fat hummus and filled with sliced salad vegetables or sweet peppers and maybe a handful of fresh beansprouts. Nice with a mug of hot miso soup or low-calorie slim soup.

- Fatoush (page 126) with 50g cubed half-fat mozzarella or 3–4 tablespoons canned chickpeas.
- Stir-steam of Vegetables (page 121) for a weekend lunch.
- Soufflé Omelette (page 101) if at home. At work, Mashed Red Bean and Soft Cheese Sandwich (page 97).

MAIN COURSES

- Oh So Simple Spaghetti and Mushrooms (page 115). Dessert: 1 low-fat fruit fromage frais sprinkled with a small handful crunchy fruit cereal.
- Grilled large flat mushrooms served with a portion of Golden Roots (page 106) and microwaved spinach. Dessert: 2 sliced kiwis with a scoop of low-fat ice cream.
- Risotto to Suit (page 116) served with a crisp green salad tossed in a low-fat dressing (page 129). Dessert: 1 small handful of grapes and 1 finger (less than 50g) of Brie or Edam cheese.
- Tagine-style Vegetables and Harissa Couscous (page 111). Dessert: 2 peeled and sliced oranges sprinkled with a little grated lemon rind and chopped fresh mint.
- Lentil 'Bolognese' with Grilled Vegetables and Pasta (page 112). Dessert: bowl of sliced strawberries and slice of melon, which could be trickled with 1 tablespoon of port.
- Weekend/Saturday dinner – Thai Tofu Curry (page 108) with Thai rice noodles. Dessert: Rice Pudding (page 133) made with Thai jasmine rice and skimmed milk, plus 2 tablespoons coconut milk stirred in. Nice with sliced fresh mango.
- Sunday lunch/dinner – Vegetable Roasties with Paprika Yogurt Sauce (page 120) plus boiled green vegetables of your choice. Dessert: 2 peach halves brushed with a little melted low-fat vegetable spread, plus maple syrup or runny honey and ground cinnamon, then grilled. Served with a trickle of

single cream or low-fat yogurt and pinches of demerara sugar or a few flaked toasted almonds.

EASY PICKINGS

With the best will in the world, however well balanced your meals are, there may be a few times during the day when you feel the need to reach for 'a little something' to nibble. This is where danger can lie in wait because packs of high-fat snacks scream at us from supermarket shelves and are easy to lay in store. Often, particularly if you have a family to feed and are juggling to coincide mealtimes, it could be a question of having to wait an hour or so until you can all sit down together. It is easy to eat properly when you are on your own, but not so easy when there are others to take into consideration.

One solution is to recognize the fact that you do like a biscuit or two (or whatever) and get in low-fat or lite versions. Oatcakes and rich tea biscuits are slightly higher in fat but good for a treat and for dunking into tea or coffee.

Instead of digestive biscuits, buy packs of **rice cakes.** Instead of chocolate bars, try a **banana, carrots** or **sweet, just ripe, juicy pears**.

In place of biscuits or crisps try: **grissini sticks, water biscuits, rice cakes** and **cream crackers**.

Fancy something sweet after a meal? Instead of reaching for the chocolate, have a small handful of naturally sweet **raisins** or 3–4 **dried apricots**.

It may be hard at first because your taste buds have to adjust, but it soon becomes second nature.

In the fridge pack a daily box of **veggie sticks** – young tender carrots, strips of sweet red pepper, sticks of mooli (white radish) and leaves of little gem lettuce. Make a **low-fat dip** with a small tub of natural yogurt, a tablespoon of 'lite' mayonnaise, a teaspoon of garlic purée (see page 83) and a shake or two of soy sauce. This is still lower in calories than a pot of even half-fat hummus. (For other dressing ideas, turn to page 129.) Dip into the box and dressing at any time of the day.

For a light, light snack, have a bowl of **salad**, which takes just minutes to put together. Shred a little gem lettuce or tear up a few iceberg leaves. Add a few slices of freshly cut cucumber, a ripe plum tomato chopped, a coarsely grated carrot and maybe some sliced radish. Tear in leaves of fresh basil or even snip over some fresh parsley or a salad onion. Sprinkle with a squeeze of fresh lemon juice and light soy sauce. If you have a batch of **home-sprouted beans** in the fridge, top with a fistful of those, even a teaspoon or more of **sunflower seeds**. It's quite amazing how such a low-calorie salad bowl can fill you up and it takes you time to chew your way through it.

Soup is a good filler. Keep it in the fridge, then when you feel the hunger pangs, heat up a mugful in a trice.

On cold days, I make a cup of instant **miso soup** served with 2 rye crackers. In fact, **soup** is a good filler, full stop. There are a number of recipes in this book that are ideal for just that purpose.

One of the popular diets at the moment is based on a big bowl of cabbage soup to which you add various other ingredients. Not a bad principle as a snack attack but not one to follow for too long. However, for the first few days of any diet it is a good idea to make a large pot of **vegetable soup** using a selection of low-calorie leafy green and root vegetables, flavouring with herbs, stock powders and soy sauce. Keep it in the fridge, then when you feel the hunger pangs, heat up a mugful in a trice. As easy as making a cup of tea.

APPENDIX

USEFUL CALORIE FIGURES

Foods are listed here in usable forms, not the more scientific 100g/100ml units that appear on packaging. This list will help you to mix and match your own meals and dishes and it also gives you an idea of what you can nibble without guilt – or binge on as a treat.

Please note that the figures are for calories (kilocalories) and are an approximate guide only.

Carbohydrates
(No added fat)

1 medium-size potato, baked or boiled, skin on (200g)	210
cooked Chinese or Japanese noodles (150g)	205
1 scone	198
10cm length French bread	196
1 croissant	185
1 pitta bread, white or wholemeal	180
soaked bulghur wheat (150g)	177
5 heaped tablespoons cooked rice (150g)	175
big fistful cooked pasta, inc. spaghetti (150g)	175
1 big fistful oven chips, reduced-fat (100g)	167
1 burger bun	140
1 wholemeal muffin	140
1 crumpet	91
1 medium slice white bread	83
1 medium slice wholemeal bread	80
1 digestive biscuit	73
1 oatcake	60
1 poppadum	53
1 rich tea biscuit	45
1 cream cracker	35
1 rye crispbread	27
1 rice cake	23
1 Scandinavian crisp roll	24
1 breadstick	21

Cereals

crunchy oat cereal (50g)	220
1 morning cereal bar	140
1 crunchy cereal bar	131
Cornflakes, Rice Krispies and Special K (30g)	111
porridge oats, 4 tablespoons (30g)	110

added-sugar muesli (30g)	106
Bran Flakes (30g)	96
All Bran (30g)	90
sugar-free muesli (30g serving)	66
Weetabix (per biscuit)	43

Dairy products

1 tub very low-fat fruit fromage frais	85
1 large egg	80
1 tablespoon double cream (48%) fat	66
milk, semi-skimmed (small glass, 125ml)	62
1 egg yolk	60
1 tablespoon crème fraiche (40% fat)	57
milk, skimmed (small glass, 125ml)	52
1 tablespoon coconut cream	32
1 tablespoon single/soured cream (18% fat)	30
1 tablespoon half-fat crème fraiche (20% fat)	25
1 tablespoon coconut milk	24
1 tablespoon Greek-style yogurt	20
1 tablespoon fromage frais (8% fat)	17
1 tablespoon low-fat natural yogurt	10
1 tablespoon fromage frais (0%) fat	8

Cheese

Stilton (50g chunk)	209
full-fat soft cheese (e.g. garlic and herb, 50g)	205
paneer Indian cheese (50g)	160
Edam, Feta and Brie cheeses (50g chunk)	157
soft goat's cheese (50g)	157
mozzarella (50g)	150
lite mozzarella (50g)	105
ricotta (50g)	92
medium-fat curd cheese (50g)	90
1 tablespoon grated mature Cheddar cheese (10 g)	40
1 tablespoon curd cheese	24
1 teaspoon freshly grated parmesan cheese (5g)	20
1 tablespoon skimmed-milk soft cheese (quark)	16
1 tablespoon virtually fat-free cottage cheese	12

Fats and oils

1 tablespoon any oil (100% fat)	120
1 teaspoon any oil (100% fat)	40
1 teaspoon butter	35
1 teaspoon olive oil spread (63% fat)	30
1 teaspoon very low-fat spread (27% fat)	26

Proteins

small can baked beans (205g)	154
4 tablespoons cooked pulses (e.g. lentils, beans)	141
1 tablespoon peanut butter	120
1/2 block firm tofu (125g)	110
1 tablespoon half-fat hummus	50
6 tablespoons reconstituted soya chunks	40

Nuts and seeds

nuts, small fistful (about 25g)	160–200
1 tablespoon unsalted peanuts	100
1 tablespoon pine nuts	100
1 tablespoon sunflower seeds	90
1 tablespoon chopped walnuts	70
1 tablespoon chopped hazelnuts	67
10 unsalted cashews	60
1 tablespoon pistachios	60
1 tablespoon flaked almonds	50
1 teaspoon sesame seeds	13
1 teaspoon poppy seeds	10

Vegetables

1/2 plantain, raw	130
1 small avocado	80
3 tablespoons sweetcorn	70
1 parsnip	70
6 olives, unstoned	70
6 tablespoons peas	50
1 leek	30
big fistful fresh beansprouts	28
1 mugful fresh spinach leaves, uncooked	26
1 medium onion, raw	25
1/2 medium-size onion	23
1 courgette	22
1 tomato	20
1 little gem lettuce	20
1 carrot	20
shredded raw cabbage, big fistful	20
1 pepper/capsicum (any colour)	20
5 tablespoons sprouts	16
1/2 small aubergine	15
small bundle green beans (1 portion size)	15
cauliflower florets, big fistful	15
1/2 head broccoli	14
6 medium-size button mushrooms	10
6 asparagus spears	10

3 radishes	10
salad cress/watercress (1 punnet or bag)	10
1 stick celery	5
$\frac{1}{2}$ cucumber	5

Fresh fruit

1 banana	100
grapes, fistful	75
1 pear	70
1 apple	60
1 fresh date	60
1 kiwi	50
1 orange	50
$\frac{1}{2}$ grapefruit	50
1 pawpaw	45
$\frac{1}{2}$ Galia melon	40
fresh strawberries, fistful	30
1 plum	20

Dried fruit and sugars

1 tablespoon hazelnut chocolate spread	85
raisins, small fistful (about 20g)	50
1 tablespoon honey	45
1 tablespoon maple syrup	39
1 tablespoon high-fruit jam	36
1 dried fig	20
1 pitted prune	16
1 teaspoon white sugar	15
1 dried apricot	12
1 teaspoon artificial sweetener	2

Dressings

1 tablespoon mayonnaise	108
1 tablespoon light mayonnaise	52
1 tablespoon vinaigrette salad dressing	40
1 tablespoon chutney	35
1 tablespoon ketchup	18
1 tablespoon tomato purée	13
1 tablespoon vinegar	0
1 tablespoon fresh lemon juice	0

Desserts

half a 500ml pot fresh cream vanilla ice cream	300
half a 500ml pot chocolate-chip ice cream	280
soft scoop vanilla ice cream, 2 scoops	180

1 choc ice	115
1 tropical fruit cocktail ice lolly	100
mango sorbet, 2 scoops	89
diet vanilla 'ice cream', 2 scoops	70
lemon sorbet, 2 scoops	70

Drinks and alcohol

440ml can lager	150
1 mug hot chocolate (2 teaspoons + 300ml skimmed milk)	150
330ml can cola	146
440ml can lite beer	120
1 glass (200ml) Florida-style orange juice	98
1 glass (200ml) clear apple juice	98
1 small glass (120ml) red wine or champagne	90
1 small glass (120ml) dry white wine	85
1 mug white coffee or tea (with milk)	12
330ml can diet cola	1.3
1 mug black coffee or tea	0

Miscellaneous

50g (½ 100g bar) dark chocolate	250
1 small apple pie	190
potato crisps (30g pack)	161
1 jam tart	140
reduced-fat crisps (30g pack)	131
1 fun-size chocolate bar	120
1 chocolate mini-roll	115
1 lower-fat chocolate bar (e.g. Flyte)	98
1 sachet instant slim soup	60
1 mint humbug	37
1 boiled sweet	20
1 teaspoon Marmite/yeast extract	13
1 sachet miso soup	9